METABOLISM OF THE NERVE TISSUE IN RELATION TO ION MOVEMENTS IN VITRO AND IN SITU

SLOVAK ACADEMY OF SCIENCES

INSTITUTE OF NORMAL AND PATHOLOGICAL PHYSIOLOGY

SCIENTIFIC EDITOR: PROF. DR. JURAJ ANTAL, DRSC.
RECENSENT: DOC. DR. VILIAM MÉZEŠ, CSC.

TRANSLATED BY DR. K. OŠANCOVÁ

MICHAL RUŠČÁK
AND
DAGMAR RUŠČÁKOVÁ

METABOLISM
OF THE NERVE
TISSUE IN RELATION
TO ION MOVEMENTS IN VITRO
AND IN SITU

UNIVERSITY PARK PRESS,
BALTIMORE—LONDON—TOKYO

Library of Congress Catalog Card No. 73-171235

ISBN 0-8391-0031-0

PUBLISHING HOUSE OF THE
SLOVAK ACADEMY OF SCIENCES,
CZECHOSLOVAKIA, BRATISLAVA 1971
Exclusive distributors for non-Socialist territories:
UNIVERSITY PARK PRESS,
115 CHAMBER OF COMMERCE BUILD.,
BALTIMORE, MARYLAND 21202, USA

CONTENTS

INTRODUCTION

In investigations of the metabolism of the CNS its morphological heterogeneity as well as the close integration of metabolic processes in relation to structure and function must be taken into account. Studies of the liver metabolism, the function of which is predominantly biochemical in nature, are quite different from the CNS in regard to organ function, the main role of which is coordination of organ functions and relations of the macroorganism to its environment, whereby the metabolism of the nervous tissue is only the basis on which this regulating function of the nervous system is effectuated.

When the relationships of the function and metabolism of the CNS are investigated its morphological heterogeneity and fine structure must be considered first of all. This fact is important because, while in the live ca 70 % of the total number of nuclei belong to cells of the liver parenchyma, nerve cells which are the carriers of integrating functions of the CNS have, in the entire brain, only ca 5 % nuclei (Waelsch 1959), and in the cerebral cortex nerve cells represent only ca 17−20 % of the total number of cells (Heller and Elliot 1955, Nurnberger 1958). The functional, morphological, and probably also the metabolic heterogeneity of the nerve cells render a correlation between metabolism and function in the nervous tissue more difficult. Another morphological peculiarity of the structure of the CNS is its ultrastructure. While in other tissues it is possible to prove by electronoptic methods the existence of an extracellular space which amounts to about 20 % of the total volume of tissue, it is maintained that in the CNS the extracellular space is negligible (ca 5 % of the total volume) and that it is limited only to intercellular clefts with an average of 150−200Å (Luse 1956, Schultz, Maynard and Pease 1957). The spaces between capillaries and nerve cells are filled with neuropile, represented by neuron processes, synapses and a mass of glial cells and their processes wedged between the vascular system and neurons (Maynard, Schultz and Pease 1957, Hager 1964, Torack 1965). The glia is supposed to be responsible for the so-called hematoencephalic barrier, i. e. a special exchange and transport of substances between nerve cells and the circulation (Katzmann 1961, de Robertis 1965) and for maintaining the ionic balance between the neuron and its medium (Hertz 1966). Evidence for this function of the glia is provided by several facts. It has been proved that the astroglial processes cover as much as 85 % of the capillary surface (Maynard, Schultz and Pease 1957, de Robertis 1965) and from these findings the conclusion is drawn that the movements of substances between the capillaries and neurons must take place predominantly via the glia (fig. 1). The high sodium content in astroglia (Katzmann 1961, Koch, Rank and Newman 1962, Hartmann 1966) and the activation of enzymes of the oxidative cycle in the astroglia *in vitro* in tissue cultures with a sodium content higher than that in the extracellular fluid (Friede 1964, 1965), found primarily in the processes of the astrocytes, lead to the assumption that glial cells *in toto* represent a special compartment homologous with the extracellular space of other tissues (Schultz, Maynard and Pease 1957, Friede 1964, Hager 1964, de Robertis

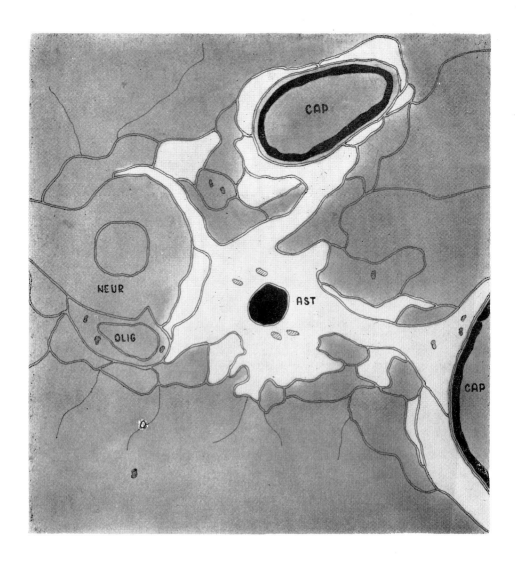

Fig. 1. Schematic diagram showing the position of astroglial cell between the capillary and the neuron. CAP—capillary, NEU—neuron, S—synapse, OLIG—oligodendroglia. AST—Astroglia. According to the concept of de Robertis.

10

1965, Hertz 1966). There are even some who believe that the glia is not only concerned with the active selection of substances between the neuron and circulation but that it also processes materials into suitable chemical forms which can serve as energy substrates for nerve cells (Hydén 1960).

Although electronmicroscopic observations rule out the existence of a greater extracellular space in the CNS, there are some serious reservations against this view. If we anticipate the transport function of the glia in the CNS, we must also assume special carriers for different substances between capillaries and glial processes on the one hand and neurons and glial processes on the other hand, whereby the transport function of the membrane on both poles of the glial cell would have to be strictly specialized, i. e. at one pole activated by a certain substance from the outside and on the other pole from the inside of the membrane. The membrane carriers would have to be in a close relationship to the formation and release of energy needed for the transport processes; this association cannot be ruled out but has not been proved so far (Kuffler and Nicholls 1966). Moreover, there is another serious point regarding the electronmicroscopic evaluation of the extracellular space in the CNS: during the fixation and dehydration a shift of ions and water occurs from the extracellular space into the cells. On the other hand, after embedding tissue into synthetic polymers their volume increases, i. e. also the volume of the embedded preparation, and this is again at the expense of the extracellular space; thus the resulting extracellular space found under the electron microscope is reduced only to narrow intercellular clefts $150-200$ Å in size which are actually found in ultrathin sections (Torack 1965). This view is supported by the work of van Harreveld et al. (1964, 1965, 1967) where evidence is provided that by a suitable fixation method, which prevents post mortem shifts of fluid and ions in the brain, and also by electronoptic methods, an approximately equal extracellular space is found as in other tissues. The fact that in the CNS by means of a suitable method Na^+ but not K^+ can be washed out also provides evidence that in the intact brain there is actually a greater extracellular space and that the exchange between cells and blood takes a similar course as in other tissues in the system: blood — extracellular fluid — cell (Kuffler and Nicholls 1966).

Not even chemical methods for the assessment of the extracellular space give an unequivocal answer. While based on the estimation of the chloride space (Tower 1958a) and the measurement of the electric conductivity (van Harreveld and Ochs 1956), it is maintained that the extracellular space accounts for about 25 % of the total mass of nervous tissue; by estimations with ^{35}S- labelled sulfate (Woodbury 1958), ^{14}C sucrose (Reed and Woodbury 1960) and ^{35}S thiocyanate resp. (Streicker 1961) evidence was provided of a substantially smaller extracellular volume which varies in nervous tissue within a range from $5-15$ % corresponding roughly to the electronoptic observations. We must therefore take into account the electronoptic findings and assume that the interrelations between glia and neuron are of decisive importance for the metabolism of nervous tissue.

Another important problem in investigations of the metabolism of nervous tissue is to determine the mutual ratio of neurons and non-neuronal cells in metabolism in relation to the tissue as a whole. Basically the given problem can be approached in three ways. If we know the ratio of nerve and non-nerve cells in different structures of the CNS, we can calculate the O_2 consumption and thus also the total metabolism of one nerve cell and non-nerve cells. From differences in the metabolism of white and gray matter of the CNS and from comparison with benign tumors the metabolic level of neurons and non-nerve cells was first calculated and the value per cell was worked out. Although it is known that there are marked differences in the morphological structure and relative representation of non-nerve cells in the gray and white matter and benign tumors resp., it proved possible, based on investigations of these structurally different components, to provide evidence that as compared with non-nerve cells the neuron has a metabolic rate of a higher order (Heller and Elliot 1955). This finding was later confirmed by other authors who worked with isolated perinuclear zones of neurons and glia (Korey and Orchen 1959) or with isolated Betz' cells and neuropile of the cortex (Epstein and O'Connor 1965, Hertz 1966). The advantage of the later findings is that they use morphologically defined structures, in particular as far as nerve cells are concerned. On the other hand, even this method has some shortcomings. Above all it works with cells which during processing are separated from their processes and glia. Thus the original relationship between glia and neuron, which only in their mutual association can be considered as a functional unit, is impaired (Hydén 1960, Hertz 1965); the structure of the cell membrane becomes less distinct or disappears altogether (Roots and Johnston 1964, Johnston and Roots 1965, Rose 1967). On the other hand, the O_2 consumption by the glial cell is not taken as a measure of the metabolism of the glia itself but rather as the metabolism of the neuropile as a whole, containing in addition to glia also dendrites and synapses of neurons, which according to Hydén (1960) have a very intense metabolic rate; therefore the findings may be strongly influenced by this fact. Work with isolated nerve cells and glia confirmed, however, the conclusions of Heller and Elliot's results (1955) that the metabolism of one nerve cell is of a higher order than that of one non-nerve cell.

Rose (1967) isolated from homogenates of the cerebral cortex by centrifuging through a density gradient two fractions, one of which contained predominantly nerve cells and the other one glial cells (neuronal-enriched and glial-enriched fraction). When he compared the O_2 consumption of these two fractions and expressed it per amount of protein, he obtained opposite results: he found practically no differences in the metabolism of glial and nerve cells.

If we consider, however, the results of the majority of authors it seems more than probable that one nerve cell has an O_2 consumption of higher order as compared with that of the non-nerve element. In view of the volume of neurons and non-nerve cells the O_2 consumption of a certain volume of neurons is $4-6$ times higher than that of neuropile (Hertz 1966) and roughly corresponds to the O_2 consumption of one liver cell.

Experiments *in vitro* have shown that a substantial portion of the energy formed by nervous tissue is used for active ion transport and the maintenance of its polarity (Gonda and Quastel 1962, Whittam 1964, Ruščák and Whittam 1967).

The high metabolic level in nervous tissue found *in vitro* was also confirmed in experiments *in situ*. The brain, although it represents only ca 1/50 of the total body-weight, utilizes as much as 1/5 of the total O_2 consumption of the organism. Determination of the arteriovenous differences revealed that the brain, even at so-called physiological conditions without interference from outside, utilizes a considerable amount of glucose; this amount is further increased during excitation. Approximately 90 % of the glucose, as apparent from the RQ which is ca 1, is oxidized to CO_2 and H_2O and about 10 % is transformed into lactate, the level of which is as a rule higher in the blood leaving the brain (Gibbs et al. 1942, Erbslöh, Klärner and Brensmeier 1958, Prokhorova and Tupikova 1959, Geiger, Kawakita, and Barkulis 1960). Geiger's experiments (1958) with the isolated cerebral circulation of the cat proved that the brain was able to utilize only glucose supplied by the blood stream and not glucose from the cerebrospinal fluid. That glucose is essential for maintaining nervous activity is apparent also from the well known fact that when the glucose blood level drops below a certain value, seizure activity is observed which in men is associated moreover with loss of consciousness. Glucose is the only substrate which can maintain the chemical composition and reactivity of nervous tissue (McIlwain 1959).

As far as glucose metabolism in nervous tissue is concerned, it differs considerably from that in other tissues. While in all tissues except the nervous system ^{14}C glucose is transformed mainly into glycogen, lactate and CO_2, in nervous tissue *in vitro* as well as *in situ* the carbon of the glucose molecule appears already after 1 min to be used in large amounts in amino acids (Beloff-Chain et al. 1955, Geiger et al. 1958, Roberts et al. 1958, Tsukada et al. 1958, 1960, Kini and Quastel 1959, Gaitonde, Richter and Vrba 1962, Machiyama, Balázs and Julian 1965), mainly in glutamic and aspartic acid, glutamine and GABA and to a smaller extent in alanine and glycine; the transformation of fructose as compared with that of glucose is much slower. The formation of the above-mentioned amino acids from glucose is a strictly aerobic process. Under anaerobic conditions the glucose utilization was only about 10 % of the values recorded during aerobic incubation; of that amount ca 80 % of the glucose was broken down to lactate and ca 20 % was found as free intracellular glucose. If the lactate formation under aerobic and anaerobic conditions was compared, it was found that the amount of lactate produced under aerobic conditions was as much as three times greater. Regional differences in the transformation of the ^{14}C glucose chain into amino acids were also found. While in other amino acids there was no difference between different areas of the CNS as regards the incorporation of ^{14}C glucose into amino acids, in the hypothalamus a 3−4 times higher formation of ^{14}C GABA was found than, e. g. in the cortex or cerebellum (Udenfriend, Weissbach and Mitoma 1960).

Also the composition of the amino acid pool differs from that of other tissues. Most striking is the occurrence of N-acetyl aspartic and γ-aminobutyric acid as well as a high content of dicarboxylic amino acids. The high concentration of glutamic acid and the presence of glutamic acid decarboxylase in nervous tissue only provides evidence of the key position of glutamic acid in the metabolism of the CNS. Attention to the importance of glutamic acid in the metabolism of the CNS was drawn as early as in 1938 by Weil-Malherbe who found that among a large number of tested amino acids only glutamic acid was able to maintain *in vitro* the metabolism at an equally high level as glucose. The substitution of glucose by glutamic acid was explained by Krebs' and Bellamy's (1960) experiments. The above authors incubated brain cortex slices with glutamic acid in the presence of minimum amounts of oxalacetic acid and found that glutamic acid was oxidized to aspartic acid: glutamic acid liberated by transamination with oxalacetate α-oxoglutarate, which by oxidation to oxalacetate created conditions for further transamination of glutamate to oxalacetate; an excess of aspartic acid was formed as illustrated by the following equation:

$$Glu + 1^{1}/_{2} O_2 \rightarrow Asp + CO_2 + 3 H_2O.$$

Cohen et al. (1962), however, provided evidence that aspartic acid is not formed by transamination of glutamate to oxalacetate and oxidation of glutamic acid molecule in the oxidative cycle but directly by decarboxylation of C_5 of glutamic acid.

Further light has been thrown on glutamate utilization by experiments *in situ* with insulin hypoglycemia: when the glucose supply to the brain is diminished, glutamic acid is utilized by transamination with oxalacetate (Dawson 1950, Okumura, Otsuki and Nasu 1959, Massieu et al. 1962). The same reaction is also encountered when the oxidative cycle is blocked with fluoroacetic acid at the citric acid level. In this case also glutamic acid is used as a source of energy for nervous tissue, but its amino group is transferred also to pyruvic acid (Awapara 1952, Dawson 1955). The reaction glutamate—pyruvate is in addition to the transamination glutamate—oxalacetate the second main route of glutamic acid utilization in the tricarboxylic acid cycle (Klingenberg 1963). Its importance in the metabolism of the CNS is suggested also by the fact that the activity of both mentioned reactions is (after heart and liver) the highest among all other tissues (Cohen and Hekhuis 1940).

Evidence on the utilization of glutamic acid in oxidative processes is provided by experiments with labelled ^{14}C glutamate. When ^{14}C glutamic acid was added to brain cortex slices, ca 40 % of $^{14}CO_2$ from glutamic acid was recovered. When ^{14}C glutamic acid and unlabelled glucose were used as substrates, the ratio of $^{14}CO_2$

remained the same. It is therefore concluded that glucose did not inhibit the oxidation of glutamic acid even when present in adequate amounts. On the other hand, when unlabelled glutamic acid was added to the medium, the formation of $^{14}CO_2$ from U-^{14}C glucose declined because part of CO_2 came from the glutamate molecule (Chain, Cohen and Pocchiari 1962).

The key role of glutamic acid in the metabolism of the CNS is proved also by the presence of γ-aminobutyric acid in the nervous tissue. γ-Aminobutyric acid, which is formed due to the action of the enzyme glutamate decarboxylase, is found, similarly to the enzymes producing and breaking it down, only in the gray matter of nervous tissue but not in other tissues (Albers and Brady 1959); the metabolic shunt glutamate $-\gamma$-aminobutyric acid probably plays an important role in the energy yielding processes of nervous tissue (Robinson 1959). As was demonstrated by experiments of McKhann and Tower (1959), cerebral mitochondria can oxidize GABA whereby the ratio of CO_2 in the total CO_2 production depends on the ratio of GABA-α-oxoglutarate present in the medium. It is assumed that in seizures due to B_6 deficiency or after administration of B_6 antivitamins the seizures are associated with reduced metabolism of the CNS at the level of the GABA shunt (Tower 1960).

A typical property of the phylogenetically higher structures of the gray matter of the CNS is the increase of the metabolism following physical or chemical stimulation. Best and longest known is the effect of potassium ions on O_2 consumption and aerobic glycolysis by cerebral cortex slices *in vitro* (Ashford and Dixon 1935, Dickens and Greville 1935, Dixon 1949, McIlwain 1959, Hertz and Schou 1962 and many others). When the potassium values in the medium where the brain cortex slices were incubated were raised above levels of the extracellular fluid, the O_2 consumption and aerobic glycolysis rose, probably as a result of a more intense ion transport across cell membranes which tried to take up more potassium from the external environment and thus to maintain their electrochemical gradient. An effect similar to the increase of external potassium was also observed following electric stimulation (McIlwain 1959).

Evidence of the increased cell membrane activity stimulating metabolism in the nerve tissue has been provided by experiments with ouabain, which selectively blocks active ion transport. When ouabain was added to tissue slices incubated in a medium with a high potassium content, the rise [of [O_2 consumption was blocked as well as the potassium transport into the cells (Gonda and Quastel 1962, Blond and Whittam 1964, Minikami, Kakinuma and Yoshikawa 1963, Ruščák and Whittam 1967 and others).

The ratio of metabolism in the active ion transport in nervous tissue amounts, depending on the animal species, to $40-70 \%$ of the total metabolism (Gonda and Quastel 1962, Blond and Whittam 1964, Minikami, Kakinuma and Joshikawa 1963, Ruščák, Ruščáková and Hager 1967, Ruščák and Whittam 1976 and others). The decisive role is played by the mutual ratio of uni- and bivalent cations as well as by the presence of sodium, which in the external environment is indispensible for the rise of metabolism associated with active ion transport.

A raised metabolism in the cortex was observed *in situ* during its stimulation with electric current or by drugs (Klein and Olsen 1947, Bain and Pollock 1949, Dawson and Richter 1949, Ruščák 1961, Carter and Stone 1962 and others), as well as during perfusion of isolated portions of the cortex with a solution containing a high potassium content (Grenell 1959).

Although it is known that the metabolism is raised in the stimulated brain cortex, the cell types of the cortex which condition this rise cannot be differentiated. According to Hertz (1965, 1966) and Wendel-Smith and Blunt (1965) the glia is responsible for the raised metabolism in stimulated tissue. If to isolated nerve cells or glia resp. in a so-called "balanced" medium (with an ion content which roughly equals that of the extracellular fluid), an excess of potassium was added, the O_2 consumption rose in preparations of glia but not in the nerve cell. On the other hand, in a sodium-free medium the O_2 consumption in the glia declined very rapidly while the CO_2 of the nerve cell was not influenced. From these experiments the conclusion has been drawn that the glia is responsible for the metabolism associated with active ion transport.

The increase of metabolism after stimulation of nervous tissue *in vitro* as well as *in situ* is mainly at the expense of glucose (Chain, Cohen and Pochriari 1962, Geiger 1958, Kini and Quastel 1959, Prokhorova and Tupikova 1959). But there too, as apparent from experiments with ^{14}C glucose, the latter is not oxidized directly but in a dynamic equilibrium with the utilized amino acids. The stimulated respiration of cortical slices with potassium in the presence of ^{14}C glucose causes a marked rise of activity in glutamine and GABA, less so in glutamate and alanine, while the activity of aspartic acid declines (Kini and Quastel 1959). As compared with non-stimulated tissue, the rise of alanine is also statistically significant (Quastel 1959). The formation of alanine rose even when $3\text{-}^{14}C$ pyruvate was used as substrate instead of glucose (Chain, Cohen and Pocchiari 1962, Beloff-Chain et al. 1962).

The utilization of non-carbohydrate components, in addition to glucose, is described by Geiger (1958) in experiments *in situ*. When he administered pentamethylene tetrazole to cats with extracorporeal brain circulation and $U\text{-}^{14}C$ glucose in the rinsing fluid or when he stimulated the cortex of the sensory-motor area with electric current or afferently via the plexus brachialis, he found that even this stimulation did not increase the production of $^{14}CO_2$, although the amount of consumed O_2 corresponded to a higher glucose uptake and thus brain had to utilize in oxidative processes also non-carbohydrate components. In several publications (Geiger 1958, Geiger et al. 1956, 1958, 1960a, b) evidence was provided that the cortex used during stimulation not only amino acids but also its own structural components, such as lipids and nucleoproteins, as a source of energy. This view is in keeping also with the findings of Ruščáková (1964a, b), who described a decrease of nucleoproteins in cortex *in situ* after stimulation by potassium or strychnine or, conversely, their enhanced formation 1−2 days after the stimulation was discontinued.

The close relationships between carbohydrate and amino acid metabolism which depend on the functional state and thus also on changes in the intra- and extracellular ionic composition in nervous tissue served as a stimulus for our own work, the results and views of which are summarized in subsequent chapters. We focused our attention on investigations of metabolic processes in the cerebral cortex *in vitro* and *in situ* in relation to the ion movements and their active transport.

METABOLISM OF NERVE AND NON-NERVE CELLS OF RAT CEREBRAL CORTEX IN VITRO

The metabolic level of nervous tissue is very high *in vitro* as well as *in situ*. The CNS, although it only accounts for ca 1/50 of the total body-weight, consumes even at so-called rest $15-20\%$ of the total amount of O_2 utilized by the organism as a whole. Estimations of the arteriovenous difference of O_2 in blood flowing through the brain have shown that 1 g of cerebral tissue consumes per minute $1.5-2\mu$ moles of O_2. Similarly, as *in vitro*, *in situ* a high O_2 consumption was also found as compared with non-excitable tissues (Elliot 1957, McIlwain 1959).

The high metabolic level and the great morphological heterogeneity of nervous tissue raised the question whether the metabolism of the CNS is a simple sum of metabolically equivalent though morphologically heterogeneous cells or whether there exist quantitative and qualitative differences between various cells of nervous tissue. So far we are unable to answer this question unequivocally because *in situ* the metabolism of the CNS as a whole is evaluated, while *in vitro* certain portions are used which are devoid of relations with the whole CNS which is a functional and morphological unit. Thus, for instance, *in vitro* the cerebellar cortex has a lower O_2 consumption than the glia from the corpus callosum and the latter has, as compared with slices of the cerebral cortex, a lower O_2 consumption although the total number of cells per volume of white as well as gray matter of these formations is approximately equal (Heller and Elliot 1955, Ridge 1967).

So far the metabolism of the cortex *in vitro* was studied in detail, i. e. its metabolism as a whole as well as that of isolated cell elements. The conclusions of experiments carried out by different authors (Heller and Elliot 1955, Korey and Orchen 1959, Epstein and O'Connor 1965, Hertz 1966, Ruščák, Ruščáková and Koníková 1967) provide evidence that neurons of the cerebral cortex have a metabolism of higher order as compared with non-nerve cells. Since, however, some work was also published stating that there are no differences in the metabolism of neurons and the glia (Rose 1967, Bradford and Rose 1967), we devoted part of our work to problems of the metabolism of nerve and non-nerve elements of the cerebral cortex in rats. Contrary to hitherto used procedures where the metabolism of neurons and non-nerve cells of the cortex was compared by confronting metabolic properties of the white and gray matter (Heller and Elliot 1955) and of isolated nerve and glial cells resp. (Korey and Orchen 1959, Epstein and O'Connor 1965, Hertz 1966, Rose 1967, Bradford and Rose 1967), we selected in our investigation a different procedure. By mechanical lesion of a part of the cerebral cortex the number of the nerve cells was reduced, whereby, however, the non-nerve cells remained preserved except for certain histological changes; based on metabolic differences of intact cortex and cortex with a relative predominance of non-nerve cells we were able to assess approximately the metabolism of one neuron and one non-nerve cell. We assume that this experimental procedure was less drastic than the isolation of nerve and glial cells, because it is known that in the course of isolation the outlines of cell membranes disappear (Roots and Johnston 1964, Johnston and Roots 1965).

Our procedure was as follows: When removing the skull bones above the convexities of both hemispheres we inserted a needle (diameter 0.40 mm) parallel with the surface of the cortex 18 times to an average depth of 4.5 mm and allowed the animals to survive for 8, 15 and 30 days; then the animals were used for experiments. From the convexity of the hemispheres freehand slices of the cortex were prepared (the left cortex from the same animal served as a control), incubated in Krebs-Ringer phosphate solution with 6.6 − 10 mM glucose after one hour in an O_2 atmosphere and the O_2 consumption was followed up. Cajal's gold-sublimate impregnation of astrocytes was used and the zone of disappeared nerve cells was measured on sections perpendicular to the inserted needle by means of an objective micrometer.

As is apparent from fig. 2, in the surrounding area of insertion into the cortex the nerve cells disappeared and their place was taken by hypertrophic glia. It may be assumed from the reaction observed that the insertion of the needle into the cortex caused smaller direct damage of tissue than the diameter of the needle itself, and that the main reason for the destruction of the nerve cells was the increased pressure in the vicinity of the needle to which nerve cells, contrary to non-nerve elements, are extremely sensitive. By multiplying the area of the circle without neurons by the number of insertions and their depth we obtained the entire statistical volume of the cortex lacking nerve cells; this amounted in our experiments to 15.6 mm³ which was ca 20 % of the total weight of tissue used for the experiment (80 mg) (Ruščák, Ruščáková and Hager 1967).

The determination of the total nitrogen in the intact cortex and cortex with a predominance of glia did not show any differences (2.06 and 2.03 g resp.) in 100 g wet wt, similarly as the dry weight content (20.5 and 20.3 % resp.).

As apparent from the data given in table 1, in the cortex with a relative predominance of glia the O_2 consumption decreased, as compared with that of the intact cortex. This drop was observed from the very onset of incubation and was also found 15 or

Table 1

	C		E
I	90 ± 3.2	$n = 15$ $P < 0.01$	78 ± 2.3
II	90 ± 4.2	$n = 12$ $P < 0.05$	79 ± 2.7
III	94 ± 4	$n = 12$ $P < 0.02$	81 ± 2

Oxygen consumption in μmoles (M ± S. E. M.) /g wet wt/hr in rat brain cortex slices of control (C) and experimental hemispheres with relative predominance of non-neuronal elements (E) after 8, (I), 15 (II) and 30 (III) days following partial mechanical lesion of the cortex. 5 mM K⁺ in the Krebs-Ringer phosphate medium, substrate 6.6 mM glucose. n — number of experiments.

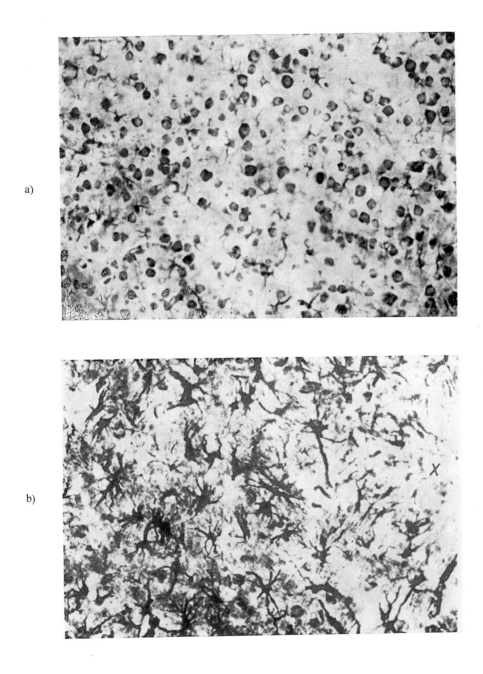

a)

b)

Fig. 2. a) Intact rat brain cortex. b) Hypertrophic astrocytes around the brain cortex lesion (X). Gold–sublimate impregnation according to Cajal.

30 days following mechanical lesion of the cortex. The potassium content was also lower in the cortex with a reduced number of nerve cells after 1 hr of incubation, i. e. 47 ± 1.6 μequiv/g wet wt as compared with 55 ± 1.8 μequiv/g wet wt of control cortex ($n = 8$, $P < 0.02$), although before incubation no differences in the potassium content between the control and experimental hemisphere were observed (108 and 106 μequiv/g wet wt resp.). The differences between the control and experimental hemispheres disappeared when the sodium in the medium was replaced by choline chloride. In this case the average O_2 consumption in the control and experimental hemispheres declined to 29 and 32 μmoles/g wet wt/hr resp.

Similar results as with the cerebral cortex of rats were obtained in cortical slices of rabbits with a relative predominance of glia cells. In the latter the O_2 consumption decreased from an average level of 60 ± 2 to 52 ± 2.6 μmoles O_2 g/hr ($n = 6$, $P < 0.05$) in a medium with 5 mM of external potassium.

Our results have shown that the cortex of rats with approximately 20 % reduced number of nerve cells *in vitro* had an O_2 consumption lower by as much as 12 μmoles O_2/g/hr, as compared with that of the intact brain cortex. Based on this difference, we calculated the approximate statistical value of O_2 consumption per nerve cell per hour in the following way: if 20 % nerve cells consume 12 μmoles O_2/g/hr, the O_2 consumption of all nerve cells will be [five times greater, i. e. 60 μmoles/g/hr. The difference $(90 - 60) - 30$ μmoles is due to non-nerve elements. From data published by Nurnberger (1958) on] the ratio of nerve and non-nerve cells in the cortex of rats we obtain for the total number of 2.17×10^7 nerve cells per 1 g cortex an O_2 consumption of 60 μmoles and for 9.7×10^7 non-nerve cells 30 μmoles: the O_2 consumption by one nerve cell then will be 6.2×10^{-5} μl O_2/hr/[1344 μl : 2.17×10^7] and that of non-nerve cell only 0.69×10^{-5} μl, [672 μl : 9.7×10^7]. The above calculations of O_2 consumption by one nerve cell are very close to the results obtained by Heller and Elliot (1955) as well as to the values reported by Korey and Orchen (1959); they are, however, lower than data reported by Epstein and O'Connor (1965) and Hertz (1966) who worked with isolated Betz' cells of the cat. If we consider, however, the fact that in our work we do not calculate the O_2 consumption per perikaryon but per cell with its processes as well as the great morphological and probably also metabolic variability of cortical nerve cells, the lower average O_2 consumption found in our experiments expressed per cell is quite conceivable.

The O_2 consumption by non-nerve elements calculated per cell was as compared with nerve cells also in our experiments, as reported in the literature (see table 2), of a lower order (Heller and Elliot 1955, Korey and Orchen 1959, Epstein and O'Connor 1963, Hertz 1966), although the absolute value in our material was lower than values reported, e. g. by Korey and Orchen (1959) or Epstein and O'Connor (1965) and Hertz (1966). The differences between the results of our experiments and data of the above authors can be explained by the fact that we used as

24

Table 2

	I	II
Heller and Elliot (1955)	$0.6 - 0.9 \times 10^{-4}$	—
Korey and Orchen (1959)	1.36×10^{-4}	1.1×10^{-5}
Epstein and O'Connor (1965)	10.2×10^{-4}	3×10^{-5}
Hertz (1966)	5×10^{-4}	0.5×10^{-5}
Own results	0.62×10^{-4}	0.69×10^{-5}

Oxygen consumption in μl O_2/hr by one neuron (I) and one non-neuronal cell (II) according to the results of various authors.

a basis findings obtained by comparing the respiration of cortical elements as a whole, while Korey and Orchen (1959) and Epstein and O'Connor (1965) and Hertz (1966) use as a basis of the O_2 consumption of non-nervous elements the respiration of isolated cells which may be contaminated by neurons, or neuropile which contains all constituents of the cortex except for the perinuclear zones of large pyramidal cells, i. e. also dendrites which are known to have a high metabolic level (Hydén 1960).

Our findings, similarly as the results of the above-mentioned authors differ from data of Rose (1967) and Bradford and Rose (1967) who did not observe any differences in the O_2 consumption between the glial-enriched fraction and the neuronal-enriched fraction which they obtained by centrifuging the cerebral cortex homogenates through a Ficoll density gradient, when they expressed the results per amount of protein and weight of tissue resp.

The unaltered dry matter and N_2 content in the control and experimental cerebral hemisphere in our material rule out the possibility that our results could be influenced by a different water content of tissue and the resulting biased calculations. We cannot maintain for certain, however, that our conclusions are free from errors because we worked with material where hypertrophy of the astroglial cells developed at the site of cortical lesion which may distort the conditions which exist in the intact cortex. We have to assume that also the O_2 consumption in the non-hypertrophic astroglia will be lower; this fact would be manifested finally by a rise of O_2 consumption by the neuron and decrease of O_2 consumption by the non-nerve cell; this emphasizes even more the finding that nerve cells have a higher O_2 consumption than non-nerve cells.

The disappearance of differences in O_2 consumption in a medium with choline chloride can be considered as evidence that the high metabolic level of nervous tissue is in a close relationship to the processes associated with active ion transport and that the latter, as also apparent from the determinations of potassium in tissue, are conditioned by the presence of nerve cells.

GLYCOGEN IN THE RAT CEREBRAL CORTEX AFTER ELIMINATION OF NERVE CELLS

Glycogen is found in the CNS in a concentration of 40−80 mg %, depending on the method of estimation and the animal species (Kerr 1936, Křivánek 1957, 1961, McIlwain 1959, Carter and Stone 1961 and others). Histochemical and electron-microscopical methods of detection revealed that in mammals glycogen is never found in nerve cells but only in the astrocytic part of the neuropile in the form of granules 200−400 Å in diameter (Friede 1954, Shimizu and Hamuro 1958, Oksche 1961, Giacobini 1964, Maxwell and Kruger 1965, Miquel and Haymaker 1965, Hager et al. 1967 and others). The occurrence of glycogen in the astroglia led to the assumption that the latter ensures the transport of carbohydrates between blood and neurons and serves at the same time as their reservoir (Oksche 1958, 1961). Since we found a lower oxidative metabolism in the cortex with a reduced nerve cell number *in vitro* it could be expected that this phenomenon will be reflected also in the amount of tissue carbohydrates *in situ*, when the supply of glucose via circulation remained unchanged.

Glycogen and glucose in the cerebral cortex were estimated enzymatically by means of the glucose oxidase test (Boehringer) after previous precipitation of glycogen according to Kerr (1936) and its hydrolysis with 1N HCl for 1 hr at 100 °C after fixation of the heads of the animals in liquid nitrogen. The tissue for histochemical analysis was fixed in Rossmann's fluid and glycogen was stained according to Bauer; for electronmicroscopic examinations the tissue was fixed *in situ* by perfusion with a 6.5 % buffered glutaraldehyde solution and postfixation of the excised tissue was completed with a 1 % solution of OsO_4. After embedding in Epon 812 the ultrathin sections were treated with lead citrate (Reynolds 1963).

Already 24 hours after a partial lesion of the brain cortex a rise in glycogen was observed which was also found 8, 15 and 30 days following the operation. On the other hand, 30 minutes after the described treatment of the cortex, we found a drop in glycogen by as much as 54 % as compared with the results of the control hemispheres (i. e. always the contralateral hemispheres of the same animal). At the same time intervals the glucose level remained unchanged, as apparent from data summarized in table 3. If in evaluation of the results the fact is considered that the shorter

Table 3

	I		II		III		IV	
	C	E	C	E	C	E	C	E
Glyc	182 ± 5.3	82 ± 9.7	190 ± 6.6	224 ± 6.6	177 ± 5	219 ± 7.2	200 ± 7.9	230 ± 9.8
	$P < 0.01$		$P < 0.01$		$P < 0.01$		$P < 0.05$	
Glc	166 ± 6	182 ± 7.4	174 ± 6	181 ± 8	—	—	185 ± 8.2	203 ± 10.6
	n. s.		n. s.				n. s.	

Glycogen (Glyc) and glucose (Glc) levels in μmoles as M ± S. E. M./g N_2 in the control (C) and experimental rat brain cortex with relative predominance of non-nerve cells (E) 30 min (I), 8 (II), 15 (III), and 30 days (IV) after brain cortex lesion. Mean values of 8 experiments. n. s. − differences statistically not significant.

the period which elapsed between the operation and the analysis of samples the higher was the content of extravasates which formed an inactive component of the analyzed tissue, the conclusion can be drawn that with the period of survival the glycogen declined in relation to the mass of analyzed tissue.

In the histochemical picture a rise in glycogen granules near the area of the lesion was found, this increase being perivascular (fig. 3a) or in the form of diffusely dispersed granules in the intercellular substance (fig. 3b). The electronmicroscopic findings revealed that glycogen accumulated only in the cytoplasm of reactively altered astrocytes of the peritraumatic area as well as in the pericapillary processes (fig. 4) and the perinuclear zone (fig. 5) and in the processes of the astrocytic cytoplasm

a)

b)

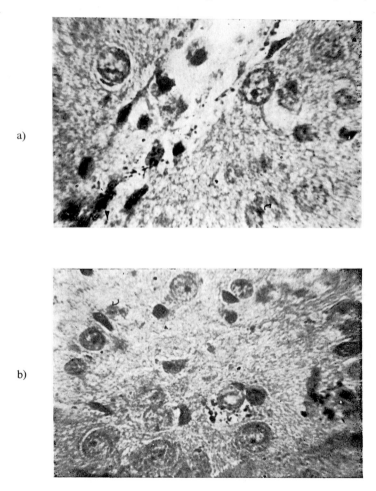

Fig. 3. PAS–positive granules in the area of hypertrophic astrocytes close to a blood vessel (a) and dispersed in the neuropile (b).

which adheres by its surface to the cell membrane of the yet preserved nerve cells (fig. 6) in form of irregularly arranged granules measuring 150—400 Å.

According to data in the literature nervous tissue accumulates glycogen when it is damaged mechanically (Shimizu and Hamuro 1958, Hager 1964, Hager et al. 1967) or by radiation (Klatzo, Miquel and Haymaker 1962, Wolfe et al. 1962, Miquel et al. 1963, Maxwell and Kruger 1965, Miquel and Haymaker 1965). It is assumed that the reason for an enhanced deposition of glycogen is either the reduced utilization of carbohydrates as a result of lowered oxidative processes in tissue with reactive astrocytes (Friede 1965, Maxwell and Kruger 1965, Miquel and Haymaker 1965, Shimizu and Hamuro 1958), or pinocytosis (Miquel and Haymaker 1965). In our opinion the only reason for deposition of glycogen in astrocytic cytoplasm of the peritraumatic area is altered interrelations in the system glia—neuron. The elimination of the neuron from this relationship leads to a decline of oxidative processes in the tissue (Ruščák, Ruščáková and Hager 1967) using glucose supplied by the bloodstream as the main source of energy (Prokhorova and Tupikova 1959). Thus although the glucose supply to the tissue by the astroglia remains the same, less of it is used in metabolic processes and therefore before the establishment of a new steady state non-metabolized glucose is partly deposited in the astroglia in form of glycogen (Ruščák, Ruščáková and Hager 1967) with a low turnover rate. This view is supported also by our experiments quoted in subsequent chapters where we found a rise of glycogen in the astroglia of the cerebral cortex after application of KCl solutions which markedly altered the structure of neurons and their oxidative metabolism.

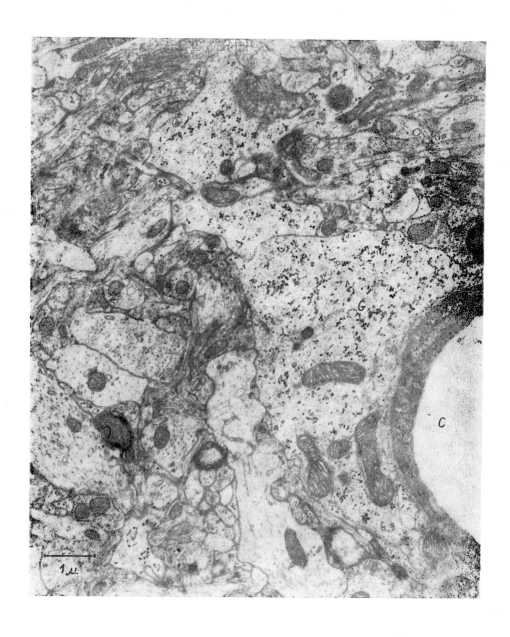

Fig. 4. Glycogen granules (G) in the end-feet of a reactive astrocyte. C — capillary.

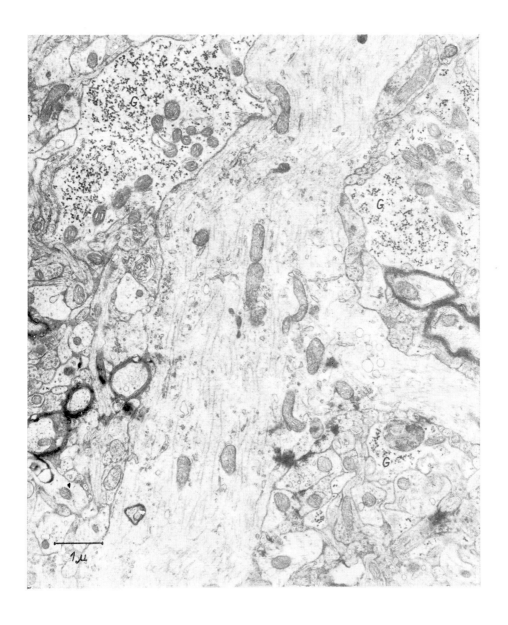

Fig. 5. Glycogen granules (G) in astroglial cytoplasm in the neuropile.

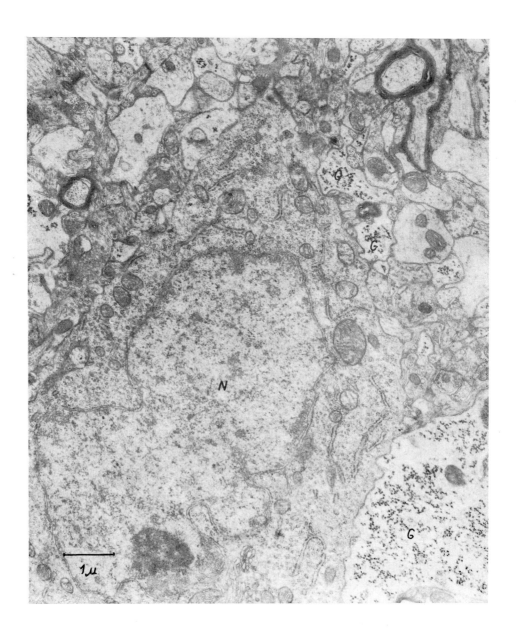

Fig. 6. Glycogen granules (G) in the perinuclear cytoplasm of a reactive astrocyte. N — neuron.

REGULATION OF BRAIN CORTEX METABOLISM IN VITRO IN RELATION TO CHANGES OF THE IONIC EQUILIBRIUM

Many experiments suggest that cell membranes of nerve tissue are involved in the regulation of its metabolic processes: slices of the cortex incubated in Krebs-Ringer phosphate solution at 0 °C lose their potassium which is replaced by sodium. If, however, the slices which lost potassium were incubated in the same solution with a suitable substrate and temperature in an [atmosphere of O_2, they gradually lost intracellular sodium which was replaced by potassium; the energy released in oxidative processes was partly used for Na^+ and K^+ transport against their electrochemical gradients (Elliot and Bilodeau 1962). Potassium added to the medium in concentrations high above the values of extracellular fluid led under the same experimental conditions to a further rise of the metabolism by ca 60 % and at the same time the potassium concentration in the cells rose at the expense of sodium (Blond and Whittam 1964). This additive stimulating effect of potassium is not observed in non-excitable tissues nor in the cerebral cortex when its morphological integrity was destroyed by homogenizing. Another peculiar feature of the cerebral cortex is that its metabolism is influenced by bivalent cations and their mutual ratio in the medium resp. Ca^{++} reduces the O_2 consumption of tissue slices in a medium with a low potassium content (5 mM) but stimulates it when the external potassium is raised above the level of extracellular fluid (Krebs 1950, Hertz and Schou 1962). The stimulating effect of calcium can be blocked by an excess of Mg^{++} ions (Hertz and Schou 1962). Because calcium is an important factor which influences the passage of Na^+ across the excitable membrane into the cell (Frankenhauser and Hodgkin 1957, Rothstein 1968), it must be assumed that its above-mentioned metabolic effects are closely related with processes taking place on the membranes. The increased metabolism in brain cortex tissue slices only in the presence of ouabain and calcium is further evidence of the participation of calcium in the regulation of the cell metabolism, depending on membrane phenomena (Schwartz 1962, Gonda and Quastel 1962).

All hitherto-mentioned metabolic effects of K^+ and Ca^{++} ions have a common feature: they all depend on the presence of Na^+ in the external medium and are associated with different rates of movement of sodium and potassium across the cell membrane by the mechanism of the sodium pump; and as the sodium pump is the factor determining the intensity of metabolism in intact cells (Judah and Ahmed 1964, Whittam 1964), we also tried to test the validity of this conclusion in slices of the brain cortex under conditions which facilitate or inhibit the sodium pump. Simultaneously we wanted to test on which type of cells the metabolic response of the cerebral cortex depends in relation to the active ion transport across the cell membrane.

In this chapter we are presenting results obtained with brain cortex slices of rabbits and rats. The tissue slices were incubated in Krebs-Ringer phosphate solution for 1 hr in an atmosphere of O_2 with 10 mM glucose as substrate. In some of the experiments the sodium in the medium was replaced by an equivalent amount of choline chloride. After the incubation was completed, the tissue filtered on muslin was dried on filter paper and in the extracts with 0.1 N HNO_3 potassium was estimated by flame photometry. The supernatant was deproteinized with $HClO_4$, final concentration 1 N, neutralized to a weakly alkaline reaction with KOH, made up to 10 ml and in a neutral solution lactic acid was determined enzymatically (Hohorst, Kreutz and Bücher 1959), or colorimetrically (Barker and Summerson 1941). All results were evaluated by means of the t-test and the results are presented as M $\pm$ S. E. M. per gram wet weight.

It was revealed, similarly as in experiments of other authors (Krebs 1950, Hertz and Schou 1962), that the omission of Ca^{++} in the medium led in a medium containing 5 mM potassium to an increase in the O_2 consumption by 30 % and a rise in the aerobic lactate formation by as much as 64 %. Already at a concentration of 0.1 mM the inhibitory effect of calcium on respiration and glycolysis were manifested. In a medium containing 5 mM K^+ the potassium content in the tissues was not influenced by a calcium-free medium and was about 10 times higher than in the medium. Because the potassium rose significantly in the tissue slices during incubation, and as it is known that the sodium pump transports potassium against a concentration gradient into the cells, it is obvious that the latter was not inhibited by the absence of calcium.

Calcium also stimulated the O_2 consumption and glycolysis in the presence of 20 μM ouabain and 105 mM potassium resp. in the incubation medium (table 4).

The experiments with tissue slices from rats with a predominance of non-nerve cells have shown that the omission of Ca^{++} from the medium stimulated the O_2 consumption as well as aerobic glycolysis in dependence on the presence of neurons. While the O_2 consumption by the intact cortex was 130 $\pm$ 4.7, in the cortex with hypertrophic glia it was only 116 $\pm$ 4.2 μmoles $O_2/g/$ hr and the rise of lactic acid was lower by 4 μmoles/g/hr after 1 hr incubation (38 $\pm$ 1.6, as compared with 34 $\pm$ 0.9 μmoles/g; $n = 8$, P close to 0.05).

Table 4

	Ca++ free Ringer						Solution with 3 mM CaCl$_2$					
	O_2	n	LA	n	K^+	n	O_2	n	LA	n	K^+	n
Control +	75 ± 3	7	39.3 ± 5.3	8	47.9 ± 1.3	11	57 ± 2.2	7	24 ± 2.6	13	47.5 ± 1.2	15
+ ouabain	45 ± 2.7	7	41.1 ± 4.2	4	13 ± 1	8	69 ± 3.5	7	34.5 ± 3	9	12.1 ± 0.1	11
+ 0.1 M KCl	82 ± 3	12	91.2 ± 5.8	7	—		96 ± 3.2	15	112.5 ± 3.5	7	—	
+0.1 M KCl + + ouabain	45 ± 3	3	91.7 ± 1.5	3	—		68 ± 1.9	6	114.4 ± 4	3	—	

Oxygen consumption (O_2) and lactate formation (LA) in μmoles as M $\pm$ S.E.M./g wet wt and tissue potassium content (K^+) in μequiv/g wet wt in rabbit brain cortex slices following 1 hr incubation in Krebs-Ringer phosphate medium with 10 mM glucose as substrate. n — number of experiments. Ouabain concentration 20 μM.

The raised O_2 consumption in a calcium-free medium led to the assumption that it may also influence the metabolic response of the cortex to inhibition of the sodium pump by ouabain. When tissue slices were incubated in a medium with 3 mM Ca^{++}, the K^+ content of the slices increased from the initial level of 25 μequiv/g to 48 μequiv/g after 1 hour's incubation. When ouabain was added in a concentration of 20 μM, to the medium with 3 mM Ca^{++}, the K^+ content in the tissue fell to 12 – 13 μequiv/g. At the same time, contrary to the calcium-free medium, the O_2 consumption by the slices in the medium with ouabain increased (for summarized results see table 4).

The graphically presented O_2 consumption (fig. 7) during incubation shows that

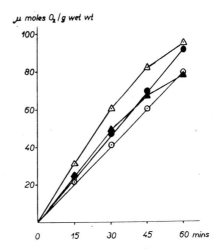

Fig. 7. Oxygen consumption by the intact rat brain cortex (●—●), by the same in the presence of ouabain (△—△), by the cortex with relative predominance of non-nerve cells (⊙—⊙) and by the same cortex in the presence of ouabain (▲—▲).

while the O_2 consumption in the medium without ouabain was linear throughout the period of incubation, a higher O_2 consumption in a medium with Ca^{++} and ouabain was found, as compared with controls, only during the first 30 min; after this period there was a marked decrease of O_2 consumption. In the calcium-free medium ouabain caused a decrease of the O_2 consumption from the very beginning of incubation. These results indicate that ouabain and calcium act together to cause a transient rise of O_2 consumption whereas singly each leads to a decrease of the metabolism of cortical slices.

Experiments with tissue slices of rats, where a relative increase of non-nerve cells was achieved by the method described in the previous chapter, have shown that the synergist influence of calcium and ouabain is bound to nerve cells because the absolute increase of the O_2 consumption by tissue slices with a predominance of glia was lower than in the intact cortex and its relative increase in relation to the results of control experiments corresponded to the decrease of the nerve cell number

39

in the experimental cortex (fig. 7). Calcium already at a concentration of 0.1 mM istimulated the O_2 consumption in the presence of 20 μM ouabain.

When in a medium with calcium or without calcium the external potassium is raised to 105 mM, both O_2 consumption and aerobic glycolysis increase. Potassium-stimulated O_2 consumption was, however, dependent on calcium ions; in their presence absolute as well as relative values were higher than in a calcium-free medium, while in non-stimulated tissue calcium had a reverse effect (table 4).

Similarly as the ouabain-stimulated O_2 consumption, the raised O_2 consumption during potassium-induced depolarization is also bound to nerve cells. The results of our experiments with tissue slices containing a relatively higher amount of non-nerve cells revealed that the O_2 consumption during of 1 hr potassium stimulation was significantly lower than that of slices from the intact cerebral cortex. The results were very similar after 8, 15 and 30 days of restitution resp. after brain cortex lesion (table 5). Also the O_2 consumption of cortical slices of rabbits stimulated by potassium declined with the reduction of nerve elements, on an average from 95 to 82 μmoles/g wet wt/hr.

When ouabain was added to the medium with a high potassium content, the O_2 consumption decreased and did not rise as in the presence of an external K^+ concentration of 5 mM (table 4). With ouabain the fall of O_2 consumption at a high K^+ level was the same in a calcium-free medium as in a medium with 3 mM $CaCl_2$. The addition of 0.1 M KCl or the omission of Ca^{++} from the medium are factors that eliminate the rise of respiration after addition of ouabain.

In the presence of 105 mM K^+ neither ouabain nor calcium had any effect on aerobic glycolysis (see table 4).

From fig. 8 it is evident that in tissue with a relative predominance of non-nerve

Table 5

	C		E
I	138 ± 4.4	$n = 15$ $P < 0.01$	119 ± 4.2
II	144 ± 4.7	$n = 8$ $P < 0.01$	122 ± 4.2
III	143 ± 6	$n = 12$ $P < 0.02$	120 ± 6

Oxygen consumption in μmoles as M ± S. E. M./g wet wt/hr by the rat brain cortex slices of control (C) and experimental hemispheres with relative predominance of non-neuronal elements (E) after 8 (I), 15 (II) and 30 (III) days following partial mechanical lesion of the cortex. n — number of experiments. 105 mM KCl in the medium.

cells even in the presence of 105 mM K$^+$ the O$_2$ consumption was lower as compared with the intact control cortex regardless whether ouabain was absent or present in a concentration of 20 μM.

The effect of ouabain makes us presume that for producing the potassium effect the operation of the sodium pump is necessary. Therefore we performed further experiments in a sodium-free medium; in order to remove sodium from tissue, the

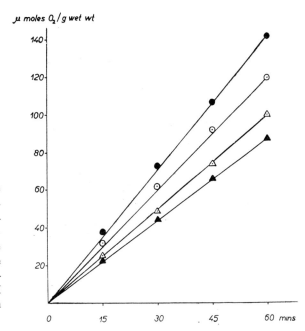

Fig. 8. Oxygen consumption by the intact rat brain cortex in the presence of 105 mM potassium (●—●) and 105 mM potassium + ouabain resp. (△—△) and by the cortex with relative predominance of non-nerve cells with 105 mM potassium (⊙—⊙) and 105 mM potassium + ouabain (▲—▲) in the medium.

slices were preincubated on ice in a medium containing choline chloride. In thus prepared slices active transport was not observed: the oxygen consumption remained at the same level, regardless of calcium, ouabain or extra potassium. It can therefore be concluded that the function of the sodium pump is indispensible for producing the above-described effects with ouabain, potassium and calcium, which are typical for the cerebral cortex.

As compared with the sodium medium, in the medium with choline chloride the lactate formation rose significantly; the latter was, however, not influenced by calcium, ouabain or extra potassium, contrary to experiments with a so-called balanced medium. From these results it is apparent that not only respiration but also glycolysis depends, due to potassium, calcium and ouabain, on the presence of sodium in the medium (for summarized results see table 6).

Oligomycin, similarly as ouabain, inhibits the activity of membrane ATP-ase associated with the sodium pump but differs from ouabain by the fact that it

41

Table 6

	Solution without Ca++						Solution with 3 mM CaCl$_2$					
	O$_2$	n	LA	n	K+	n	O$_2$	n	LA	n	K+	n
Control +	39 ± 1.4	8	62.8 ± 9	4	10.2 ± 0.2	4	36 ± 1.5	8	64.9 ± 6.7	6	7 ± 0.2	4
+ ouabain	38 ± 1.8	4	68.4 ± 4.7	4	9.0 ± 0.3	4	35 ± 2.2	6	65.3 ± 3	4	7.7 ± 0.2	4
+ 0.1 M KCl	39 ± 2.7	4	80.7 ± 3.8	4	—		36 ± 1.4	4	73.2 ± 1.4	4	—	
+ 0.1 M KCl + + ouabain	41 ± 1.2	4	93.4 ± 5.8	4	—		39 ± 2	4	77.8 ± 6.4	5	—	

Oxygen consumption (O$_2$) and lactate formation (LA) in μmoles as M ± S.E.M/g wet wt/hr and tissue potassium content (K+) in μequiv/g in the rabbit brain cortex slices incubated 1 hr in the medium in which 0.15 M NaCl was replaced by 0.15 M choline chloride. n — number of experiments. Ouabain concentration 20 μM.

reduces also oxidative phosphorylation; in view of these effects we could expect that it will influence also active ion transport. Because it is moreover maintained that oligomycin has an influence on the sodium pump elsewhere than at the ATP level (van Rossum 1964, Hempling 1966), it was important to compare its effect with ouabain about which it is known that it acts directly on membrane transport ATP-ase.

As can be seen from the summarized results presented in tables 7 and 8, oligomycin caused only a decrease of the O$_2$ consumption even when the latter was stimulated by ouabain. The production of lactate with oligomycin was always higher than with ouabain. In both of these metabolic processes the effect of oligomycin predominated over the effect of ouabain when both were present in the incubation medium. The addition or omission of calcium did not influence the O$_2$ consumption and the actate formation in the presence of oligomycin. The decrease of potassium in tissue

Table 7

	Ca++ free solution			Solution with 3 mM CaCl$_2$		
	O$_2$	LA	K+	O$_2$	LA	K+
Control +	65 ± 5	51.8 ± 2.2	46 ± 1.8	53 ± 2.4	40.9 ± 1.4	44 ± 1.4
+ oligomycin	33 ± 2.2	91 ± 9	21 ± 0.6	32 ± 1.2	89.3 ± 3.3	19 ± 0.4
+ 105 mM K+	81 ± 4.6	71.8 ± 1.6	—	90 ± 2.3	99.1 ± 7	—
+ 105 mM K+ + oligomycin	46 ± 2.7	139 ± 7.8	—	47 ± 1.4	139 ± 6.8	—

The effect of oligomycin (10 μg/ml) on the oxygen consumption (O$_2$), lactate production (LA) expressed in μmoles as M ± S. E. M./g wet wt/hr and tissue potassium content (K+) (in μequiv/g wet wt) in the rabbit brain cortex slices. Mean values of 3 experiments. Medium Krebs-Ringer phosphate, 100 % O$_2$ atmosphere, substrate — 10 mM glucose.

42

Table 8

	O_2 consumption (μmoles/g wet wt/hr)	Lactate formation (μmoles/g wet wt/hr)	Tissue K^+ content (μequiv/g)
Control +	57	33.3	55
+ 20 μM ouabain	61	49.7	12
+ oligomycin 0.5 μg/ml	42	85.1	36
+ oligomycin 1 μg/ml	42	91.9	28
+ oligomycin 10 μg/ml	40	89.2	28
+ 20 μM ouabain + + oligomycin 10 μg/ml	44	78.5	13

Different effects of ouabain and oligomycin on the metabolism of rabbit brain cortex slices. Mean values of 3 experiments. Incubation medium Krebs-Ringer phosphate + 10 mM glucose.

after oligomycin was much smaller than that after ouabain, and when both oligomycin and ouabain were added, the potassium fell to the same level as with ouabain alone.

In stimulated tissue oligomycin reduced the O_2 consumption, like ouabain, but, contrary to the former, it significantly increased the glycolysis. It can be seen from the results summarized in table 7 that oligomycin stimulated glycolysis regardless of whether the potassium content of the medium was low or high.

The effect of oligomycin depends also on the presence of sodium in the medium: if the latter was omitted, there was no difference in the metabolism of tissue, regardless of whether oligomycin or ouabain were added (table 9). The conclusion thus is that the action of oligomycin is also conditioned by the presence of sodium ions.

In order to clarify the site of action of oligomycin on active transport, we made further experiments in an atmosphere of $N_2 : CO_2 = 95 : 5$. Nervous tissue can,

Table 9

	O_2	LA	K^+
Control +	31 $\pm$ 2	65.3 $\pm$ 3.0	12.3 $\pm$ 0.6
+ oligomycin	32 $\pm$ 2.1	78.1 $\pm$ 4.1	10.9 $\pm$ 0.5
+ 105 mM K^+	30 $\pm$ 1.7	64.4 $\pm$ 6.2	—
+ 105 mM K^+ + oligomycin	28 $\pm$ 1.7	79.1 $\pm$ 2.8	—

Oxygen consumption (O_2) and lactate formation (LA) (in μmoles as M $\pm$ S. E. M./g wet wt/hr) and tissue potassium content (K^+) (in μequiv/g) in the presence of 10 μg oligomycin/ml in the medium in which NaCl was replaced by equimolar choline chloride. Mean values of 6 experiments.

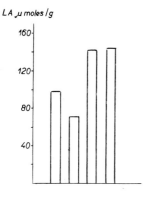

LA μ moles/g

160-

120-

80-

40-

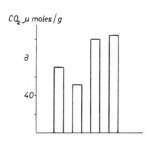

CO₂ μ moles/g

8

40-

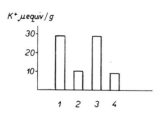

K⁺ μequiv/g

30-
20-
10-

1   2   3   4

Fig. 9. Lactic acid production (LA), CO_2 formation (CO_2) in μmoles/g wt and tissue K^+ content in μequiv/g in rabbit brain cortex slices after 1 hr anaerobic incubation in control experiments (1), in the presence of ouabain 20 μM (2), in the presence of oligomycin 10 μg/ml (3) and in the presence of oligomycin + ouabain (4).

like red blood cells, also use energy produced during glycolysis for active transport (Bilodeau and Elliot 1963); if oligomycin would influence the active transport by interfering with the activity of membrane ATP-ase, its effect would have to manifest itself also under anaerobic conditions. Our experiments showed, however, that oligomycin, contrary to ouabain, did not reduce the potassium level of tissue, as compared with controls; the tissue K^+ level was 4−5 times higher than in the medium, although in the presence of ouabain potassium declined to 10 μequiv/g. Oligomycin stimulated, however, also under anaerobic conditions the production of lactate, determined either enzymatically or on the basis of CO_2 formation. Oligomycin combined with ouabain stimulated anaerobic glycolysis but did not prevent the decrease of the potassium level in the tissue (fig. 9).

We may thus summarize that oligomycin acts as regards its effect on active transport in a different way from ouabain and its metabolic effect dominates over that of ouabain. Its interference with active transport in cortex slices is more complex than in red blood cells and its site of action is different from that of ouabain.

The results presented so far have shown that the increase of external potassium caused, as known from the work of Ashford and Dixon (1935) and Dickens and Greville (1935), a rise in the O_2 consumption and a rise in aerobic glycolysis. This response of brain cortical slices to potassium depended on the presence of sodium ions in the medium and was not encountered when the sodium pump was blocked by ouabain (Gonda and Quastel 1962, Elliot and Bilodeau 1962, Hertz and Clausen 1963). Another peculiarity of the cerebral cortex was that its metabolic response to calcium depended on the presence of Na^+ and K^+ ions in the medium. When slices were incubated in a medium with a low K^+ content (5 mM), calcium reduced the O_2 consumption and aerobic glycolysis. When, however, the potassium in the medium was raised to 105 mM, calcium in a concentration of 3 mM increased the O_2 consumption: calcium thus had a double effect on the metabolism of slices of the cerebral cortex, depending on the concentration of external potassium. A similar finding is reported by Rose (1967) who found a relationship between the O_2 consumption and the ratio of Ca^{++}/K^+ in the medium; thus Quastel and Quastel's view (1961) was confirmed that the ratio of Ca^{++}/K^+ in the medium determines the magnitude of the stimulation by potassium. Although this ratio is important, the truth remains that potassium stimulates the O_2 consumption, regardless of the presence of Ca^{++} in the medium (Elliot and Bilodeau 1962).

Calcium is closely involved in physico-chemical processes on membranes, for in excitable tissues it affects the membrane resistance, the resting and the action potentials as well as the conductivity for sodium and potassium (Huxley 1964, Rothstein 1968). However, the problem of regulation of the metabolism by calcium owing to its effect on membranes was so far not recognized. In order to contribute to the elucidation of the participation of calcium in the regulation of metabolism in relation to processes which take place on the membrane, we made experiments where we investigated its effect during elimination of the sodium pump in a choline chloride medium, or we inhibited it by means of ouabain. The results revealed that the metabolic effect of calcium was eliminated when the sodium pump was inactivated. In keeping with this finding are also those of an increased metabolism in a calcium-free medium when the permeability for sodium ions rises (Curran, Herrera and Flanigan 1963, Bolingbroke and Maizels 1959, Solomon 1960, Rothstein 1968); because the ion exchange between cells and medium is enhanced, more energy is needed to maintain the ion balance, and therefore in a calcium-free medium the metabolism is also increased.

The metabolic response to a high external potassium level and the synergistic action of calcium and potassium were conditioned by the function of the sodium pump. This effect is not observed in red blood cells, slices of the kidney cortex and liver or in homogenates of the cerebral cortex. It may therefore be concluded that the metabolic response to potassium and calcium depends on the integrity of cell membranes of excitable cells. It is probable that the increased metabolism is induced by depolarization of membranes, as was demonstrated by Hillman and McIlwain (1961) on slices of the cerebral cortex and by the subsequent increase of permeability and active sodium and potassium transport. Although experiments with the "turnover rate" of ions in slices were a failure, this assumption can be accepted with regard to results obtained with axons of marine crabs and sepia where an enhanced potassium exchange was found (Keynes and Lewis 1951, Hodgkin and Keynes 1955).

Yet another open question is the site of the ion effect. Analogously as in red blood cells and axons, it seems probable that the stimulation of metabolism by potassium is conditioned by activation of the sodium pump from outside the cell surface and that it depends on the intracellular sodium concentration (Glynn 1962,

Whittam 1962, Baker 1965, Baker and Connally 1966). The potassium effect is manifested via the sodium pump, whereby the metabolic effect is primarily regulated by the ratio $ATP/ADP + Pi$.

Despite the effect of potassium on O_2 consumption by slices of brain cortex the question remains open whether potassium enhances oxidative processes in the cortex as a whole or only in certain functionally and morphologically distinct types of cells. From our results it may be concluded that only nerve cells are responsible for the rise in the O_2 consumption by cortex slices during potassium-induced stimulation. We used as a basis the following assumption: if in the stimulated slices in our experiments the weight of tissue were reduced by 20 %, the O_2 consumption would also drop by 20 %, i. e. by 27 μmoles/g/hr. Because, however, in our experiments only the number of nerve cells declined by 20 %, we must add to this result the O_2 consumption of the remaining non-nerve cells which was, as was demonstrated earlier, 6 μmoles/hr. The thus calculated value of 117 μmoles/g/hr (138—27) is practically identical with the actually observed average 119—122 μmoles/g/hr. The above calculations indicate that while the non-nerve elements of the cerebral cortex do not respond in the same way as excitable cells, i. e. by a rise in O_2 consumption when the external potassium is raised to 105 mM, the O_2 consumption in the cerebral cortex rises only when the nerve cells are intact. The same conclusions on the relationship between potassium-stimulated O_2 consumption and nerve cells can also be drawn from experiments of Hertz and Clausen (1963) who found it only in the gray and not in the white matter. On the other hand, data of Hertz (1966) on potassium stimulation of O_2 consumption by isolated non-nerve elements are in disagreement with our results. If, however, potassium would increase the O_2 consumption by non-nerve cells in the slices independently on neurons, then we should record in our experiments in the cortex with a relative predominance of glia, as compared with intact tissue, in the medium with 105 mM K^+ a rise and not a drop in O_2 consumption. It cannot be ruled out, of course, that when the potassium level in the medium is raised, the nerve cells induce the rise in oxidative processes in glial cells; these are to represent the transport system of the neuron, and as a whole to represent the extracellular compartment of the nervous tissue supposed to condition the activity of nerve cells (Hertz 1965, Wendel-Smith and Blunt 1965); the presence of nerve cells is, however, indispensable for the stimulative effect of potassium on the O_2 consumption by cortical slices.

It is more difficult to localize the influence of calcium on metabolism than that of potassium. It seems, however, that it acts from outside the membrane. When tissue is homogenized and thus calcium gains access to the primary intracellular structures, the synergism of calcium and potassium found in slices is not encountered in homogenates (Whittam and Blond 1964). On the other hand, it was revealed that calcium inhibits the sodium pump in red blood cells from inside the membrane (Hoffman 1961, Rummel, Seifen and Baldauf 1963). It cannot be ruled out therefore that calcium acts from the outside as well as inside of the membrane of excitable cells, although there is more evidence that Ca^{++} is primarily involved in control of sodium flows from the outside of the membrane (Blaustein and Goldman 1966).

The rather unexpected finding of the synergist effect of calcium and ouabain on metabolism deserves attention as each separately always causes a drop (Whittam 1962, Schwarz 1962). As apparent from findings of a reduced K^+ content in the slices, the sodium pump was inhibited under these conditions; the O_2 consumption was, however, raised as compared with experiments without ouabain. This effect of calcium in combination with ouabain was not found in a sodium-free medium or in the presence of a high external potassium level. The described finding is difficult to interpret, as theoretically during inhibition of the sodium pump a drop in metabolism should be recorded. As the effect of ouabain in combination with calcium is not found in the liver or kidneys (Whittam and Willis 1963, Elshove and van Rossum 1963), we assume that it is specific only for the excitable nerve cells; this is suggested by our own findings as well as by data reported by Giacobini (1967), who also observed with a concentration of ouabain of the order 10^{-6} M and lower in isolated neurons of crustacea a rise in the O_2 consumption.

Oligomycin is an antibiotic that inhibits oxidative phosphorylation (Lardy Fehnson and McMurray 1958, Huijing and Slater 1961). It inhibits, however, the sodium pump in erythrocytes which do not have mitochondria, and it is therefore assumed that it can also inhibit the sodium pump in other tissues which contain mitochondria (Glynn 1963, Whittam, Wheeler and Blake 1964). For investigations of the effect of oligomycin on membrane phenomena nervous tissue is particularly suited, as it is able to maintain even under anaerobic conditions its potassium level 4–5 times higher than the potassium level of the medium. Under anaerobic conditions slices of the cerebral cortex thus should behave in a way similar to red blood cells.

Our experiments revealed, however, that the effect of oligomycin in cortical slices differs from that of ouabain and that it is much more complicated than in red blood cells. When adding oligomycin in the presence of calcium we never found a stimulation of the metabolism, as when adding ouabain, but only a drop in metabolism. Oligomycin under aerobic and anaerobic conditons always stimulated lactate production and even during maximum inhibition of the aerobic metabolism it did not block the sodium pump to the same extent as ouabain. And, finally, oligomycin, contrary to ouabain, did not influence the sodium pump under anaerobic conditions. The only common sign of oligomycin and ouabain was that their effect depended on the presence of sodium in the medium.

The mentioned facts provide evidence that the influence of oligomycin on the active transport in slices of the cerebral cortex can be interpreted only by its direct effect on the oxidative phosphorylation without postulating its direct interference with the sodium pump. It was revealed that in isolated mitochondria the ion transport is sensitive to oligomycin due to its effect on the formation of energy rich compounds other than ATP which are components in the system of oxidative phosphorylation (Chappel, Cohn and Greville 1963); however, the cellular sodium pump is not in the mitochondria but on the cell membrane and therefore further evidence is needed that the source of energy for its activity is not ATP. In our view the theory of the function of ATP in the mechanism of the sodium pump is quite sufficient. When, as a result of oligomycin, tissue respiration declines, then we can expect due to the Pasteur effect a higher lactate formation as well as a lower level of active ion transport due to a reduced ATP production.

CARBOHYDRATES OF THE CEREBRAL CORTEX IN SITU DURING DEPOLARIZATION ASSOCIATED WITH EEG DEPRESSION

Depolarization of the cerebral cortex *in vitro* is associated, as was demonstrated in the previous chapter, with a rise in the metabolism and in increased lactate production. A similar rise in the metabolism is found also *in situ* when the CNS is stimulated by electric current, drugs or in another way (Bain and Pollock 1949, Richter and Dawson 1948, Palladin 1959, Grenell 1959, Ruščák 1961 and others). A typical manifestation of stimulation of nervous tissue *in situ* is the increased carbohydrate utilization of its own reserves as well as those supplied by the blood stream and a rise of the lactate content of tissue (Prokhorova and Tupikova 1959). The disadvantage in experiments *in situ* is, however, that states of excitation cannot be defined quantitatively, although EEG activity, and thus also processes taking place on the membranes, are, no doubt, raised, as compared with intact individuals. In order to compare relationships, between the polarity of the cerebral cortex and metabolism, we selected as an experimental model Leão's spreading cortical EEG depression. The latter is described as a phenomenon in nervous tissue characterized by temporary reduction or disappearance of spontaneous and evoked electrical activity associated with depolarization which spreads from the site of elicitation at a rate of $2-3$ mm/min concentrically in the gray matter and which is preceded by a brief electrical discharge (Grafstein 1956, Marshall 1959); this process involves all layers of the cerebral cortex (Morlock, Mori and Ward jr. 1964) and its bioelectrical characteristics are identical, no matter whether it was induced by physical or chemical stimuli (Bureš 1956, Marshall 1959, Zachar and Zacharová 1963). Depolarization associated with a temporary rise in extracellular potassium (Křivánek and Bureš 1960, Brinley, Kandel and Marshall 1960), leads similarly as in experiments *in vitro* to an increased O_2 consumption (Lukyanova and Bureš 1967), to a decrease in the phosphocreatine, glycogen and glucose levels and to a rise in the lactate level of tissue (Křivánek and Bureš 1958, Zachar and Ruščák 1958, Ruščák and Duda 1959, Křivánek 1961, 1962, Ruščák 1962). The phosphocreatine level correlates closely with the polarity of tissue: its decrease precedes depolarization (Duda, Ruščák and Zachar 1961) and conversely its rise precedes repolarization (Křivánek, Bureš and Burešová 1958). From these findings it may be concluded that the polarity of the nervous tissue is closely related with the amount of $\sim$ P energy actually present in the tissue. And as nervous tissue uses almost exclusively carbohydrates as a source of energy, we focussed our attention in the first place on investigations of carbohydrates and their derivatives during depolarization caused by the EEG depression of the cerebral cortex. Contrary to Křivánek (1961, 1962), who used for analyses only depolarized parts of the cortex, we used the whole cortex of the convexity of the hemispheres. We elicited, however, the EEG depression in the cortex with a reduced blood supply after bilateral ligature of the carotid arteries. At this experimental procedure the period of negativity is protracted, as compared with intact carotid arteries, on an average $6-7$ times or more; thus we were able to use for analyses the whole cortex which was in a depolarized state.

Our experiments were as follows: under dial (Allobarbital Spofa) anesthesia (50–60 mg/kg i. p.) we made by frontoparietal sutures of both hemispheres (area 2 according to Krieg 1946, or area RAˢ according to Svetuchina 1962) trepanation openings with a diameter of 4 mm and at a distance of 2 mm another two openings with a diameter of 2 mm. The larger holes were covered with filter paper soaked in 3 M and 0.3 M KCl solution or saline and from the two small openings the EEG activity and the slow potential changes accompanying the EEG depression were recorded, using the method elaborated by Zachar and Zacharová (1963). After 30 min application of the agents causing depression of EEG activity the heads of the animals were fixed *in situ* in liquid air, the cortex of the convexity of both hemispheres was removed (cortex to which saline was applied served as control) and in the thus obtained tissue we estimated: glycogen according to Kerr (1936) as glucose after hydrolysis at 100 °C with 1 N HCl according to Somogyi-Nelson's method (1952) or enzymatically by means of the glucose-oxidase system (Boehringer), glucose, lactate (Barker and Summerson 1941), α-keto acids (Cavallini and Frontalli 1954) and citric acid (Woodbury and Vernadakis 1958). The results are presented in μmoles $\pm$ S. E. M. per g N_2, insoluble in extraction solutions and determined by microkjeldahlization; the statistical evaluation was made by the *t*-test.

It was found that depolarization of the cortex associated with depression of EEG activity was prolonged considerably during ligature of the carotid arteries as compared with intact carotid arteries (fig. 10), while the EEG activity within 30 min of the

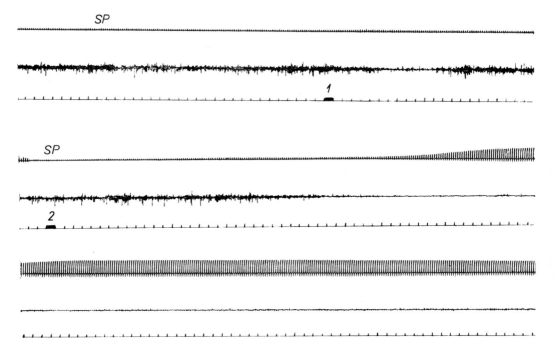

Fig. 10. Slow potential change (SP) and EEG record during spreading depression after the ligature of carotid arteries. 1 — ligated carotic arteries, 2 — to the exposed brain cortex filter paper soaked in 3 M KCl solution applied. Time — 5sec intervals.

ligature of the carotid arteries alone, after a temporary reduction in the amplitude of the EEG record, was not altered (fig. 11). Brain cortex depolarization, when the carotid arteries were ligated, led to a decrease in the glycogen and glucose content and a rise in lactate. The observed differences of glycogen and glucose were similar to those reported by Křivánek (1959, 1961, 1962) in the course of depolarization during intact cerebral circulation (the results are summarized in table 10). In the experimental cortex we found, as compared with the contralateral intact cortex of the same animal, a decrease in glycogen by 89 μmoles/g N_2, glucose by 46 μmoles/g N_2 and a rise in lactate by 280 μmoles/g N_2. Also, when the enzymatic estimations of glycogen and glucose were used, their decrease in the experimental cortex by 94 and 48 μmoles resp. per gram N_2 was found (values in controls: glycogen 189 and glucose 152 μmoles/gram N_2). While the level of keto acids was not significantly altered in the

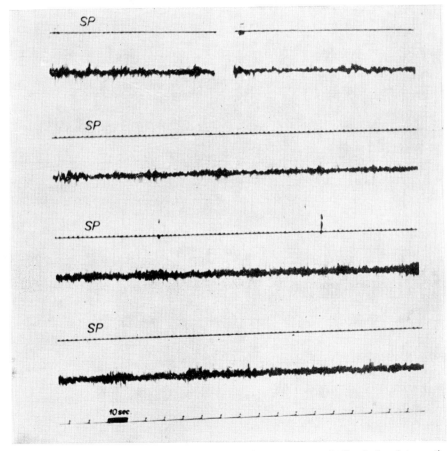

Fig. 11. Steady potential (SP) and EEG record before carotid ligature (1st line before interruption), immediately after carotid ligature (continued in the first and second lines), 15 min (the third line) and 30 min (the fourth line) after carotid ligature. Time — 10 sec intervals.

Table 10

	C	E	P
Glycogen	260 ± 17	171 ± 19	< 0.01
Glucose	190 ± 6	150 ± 5.4	< 0.01
Pyruvate	7.7 ± 0.4	6.2 ± 0.8	> 0.1
Lactate	138 ± 14	407 ± 28	< 0.01
Citrate	18.8 ± 1.1	15.5 ± 0.8	< 0.05
α-Oxoglutarate	4.3 ± 0.36	3.6 ± 0.3	> 0.1

The levels of some metabolites in the rat brain cortex expressed in μmoles as M ± S. E. M./g N_2 in the control (C) and experimental (E) hemispheres following 30 min application of 3 M KCl to the brain cortex. Ligated carotid arteries. Mean values of 10 experiments, P — statistical significance.

Table 11

	R	L
Glycogen	250 ± 15	242 ± 14
Glucose	186 ± 16	177 ± 16
Pyruvate	10.5 ± 0.9	10.2 ± 1
Lactate	139 ± 11	147 ± 13
Citrate	17 ± 0.6	18.9 ± 0.7
α-Oxoglutarate	3.9 ± 0.6	4 ± 0.7

The levels of some metabolites expressed in μmoles as M ± S. E. M./g N_2 in the right (R) and left (L) brain cortex of the same animal. Carotid arteries were ligated for 30 min. Mean values of 10 animals.

Table 12

I		II		III		IV	
C	E	C	E	C	E	C	E
138 ± 14	407 ± 28	273 ± 21	495 ± 35	476 ± 30	693 ± 45	788 ± 42	812 ± 51
$P < 0.01$		$P < 0.01$		$P < 0.01$		n. s.	

Lactic acid in μmoles as M ± S. E. M./g N_2 in the control (C) and experimental (E) rat brain cortex, to which 3 M KCl was applied for 30 min (I) and after 60 (II), 150 (III) and 240 (IV) sec of asphyxiation following compression of trachea. Ligated carotid arteries. Mean values of 10 experiments. n. s. — differences statistically not significant.

cortex to which KCl was applied, an increase in citric acid was recorded; it was, however, remarkable that we did not find detectable amounts of oxalacetic acid in our experiments. As apparent from the results of analyses of the right and left hemisphere of the same animal, no significant differences were found between them; this fact proves that the control material was well selected (table 11).

The block of external respiration leads to a drop in the polarity of the cortex which is described also as terminal anoxic depolarization. The latter developed sooner in the cortex exposed to EEG depression (Ruščák and Duda 1959) and at the same time, as evident from the data presented in table, 12 in the experimental cortex during terminal anoxic depolarization significant differences in the lactate content were found till the differences between the polarity of control and experimental cortex also disappeared after 4 min; because there was a good relationship between the increase in lactate and the decrease in glycogen and glucose, only lactate in the cortex was determined in further experiments.

The initial values were not attained 30 or 90 min restitution following the removal of applied KCl, if both carotid arteries remained ligated; on the contrary, gradually the lactate also increased in the control cortex. The differences between the control and experimental cortex remained, however, preserved. The initial state was attained only when the carotid arteries were reopened at the end of the experiment (table 13).

Similar results as with KCl were also obtained with other substances which, when applied to the cerebral cortex, caused the EEG depression (Ruščák 1962).

The decrease in the glycogen and glucose level in the cortex associated with depolarization during the EEG depression was as regards its quantitative evaluation very close to the values described by Křivánek (1959, 1961, 1962). Similarly as Křivánek's findings our experiments also showed that there was in fact a decrease in glycogen and glucose content and that the observed changes were not due to differences in the levels of substances of a non-glucose character which interfere with the estimation of glucose (Adler and Hollander 1953).

Table 13

I		II		III		IV		V	
C	E	C	E	C	E	C	E	C	E
153 ± 24	433 ± 27	160 ± 28	407 ± 38	273 ± 34	423 ± 41	148 ± 25	203 ± 21	133 ± 14	142 ± 15
$P < 0.01$		$P < 0.01$		$P < 0.01$		n. s.		n. s.	

Lactic acid in μmoles as $M \pm$ S.E.M./g N_2 in the control (C) and experimental (E) rat brain cortex to which 3 M KCl was applied for 30 min after carotid arteries ligature (I), 30 min (II) and 90 min (III) of recovery period after washing off KCl when carotid arteries were ligated and after 30 min (IV) and 90 min (V) after washing off KCl by reopened carotid arteries. Mean values of 9 experiments. n. s. — differences statistically not significant.

It was also found that the ligature of both carotids alone did not influence the level of the above metabolites in the brain. Thus for instance the glycogen level in the brain is reported to be 50—100 mg % (Kerr 1936, Křivánek 1957, McIlwain 1959, Carter and Stone 1961). If we express our results in mg %, we obtain equal values, i. e. on an average 87 mg per 100 g wet weight of cortex with the reduction method and 66 mg % with the enzymatic one (in 100 g of cortex we found on an average 1.92 g insoluble nitrogen). The glucose level was in keeping with the results which were obtained by non-specific reduction methods (Bronovickaya and Shapovalova 1957); similarly as the above authors, we found values of 55—65 mg %.

From our results we cannot tell whether the decrease in glycogen is due to its enhanced utilization or reduced formation. If we consider, however, the results of experiments *in vitro*, where excess of potassium in the external medium reduced the synthesis of glycogen and at the same time increased the utilization of glucose by tissue slices (Kleinzeller and Rybová 1957, Kini and Quastel 1959 and others), we may also assume that under our experimental conditions the decrease of glycogen in tissue was due to its increased utilization as well as reduced formation. A similar decrease in glycogen after 15 and 30 min action of KCl might suggest that in nervous tissue there is only one fraction of glycogen which is readily utilized in metabolic processes. It is possible, as assumed also by Chajkina (1959), that only glycogen not bound to constituent cell structures is used in energy processes, while glycogen bound to lipids and proteins may be a component of the structures which condition the morphological appearance of the cells.

The drop in glycogen and glucose as well as the rise in lactate can be considered the result of enhanced carbohydrate breakdown in the negative phase of the depression wave which is associated with a reduced utilization of O_2 (Lukyanova and Bureš 1967) as well as a result of diminished O_2 supply. The unaltered pyruvate level in our experiments during intense glycolysis, contrary to findings of other authors during pharmacological stimulation of the CNS (Bain and Pollock 1949, Bain, Pollock and Stein 1949), can be explained by the fact that in addition to the reduction of pyruvate to lactate its enhanced transamination with glutamic acid was also recorded, as evident from the formation of alanine which will be demonstrated in subsequent chapters. This assumption also explains the unaltered α-oxoglutaric acid level despite the fact that the increase in citric acid can indicate its slower oxidation in the tricarboxylic acid cycle.

Almost two thirds of the 6-carbon chain of carbohydrates, contrary to experiments with intact circulation, were found in the form of lactate. In our opinion this finding is due to the fact that, under conditions of a reduced blood supply to the brain and concomitant increased demands on energy associated with repolarization processes, the oxidation of reduced NADH triosephosphate dehydrogenase in the mitochondrial system of electron transport, which is supposed to be particularly intense in nervous tissue (Sacktor, Packer and Estabrook 1959, Boxer and Shonk 1960, Guminska 1961), is competitively inhibited and therefore permanent glycolysis is rendered possible only via oxidation of the reduced co-ferment of triosephosphate dehydrogenase by reduction of pyruvic to lactic acid. The inhibition of isocitric acid oxidation in the oxidative cycle, this being particularly sensitive to deficiency of electron acceptors and thus a factor regulating the equilibrium citrate/isocitrate (Kleinzeller 1954), also leads to the rise in citric acid in the experimental cortex. The unaltered level of α-oxoglutaric acid, on the other hand, provides evidence that its source under the described experimental conditions is not only the tricarboxylic acid cycle, but most probably also glutamic acid present in the CNS in concentrations which are several times higher than its blood level.

Based on hitherto described results we decided to focus our subsequent work on the elucidation of conditions determining the formation of lactate in the cortex at cellular and subcellular levels and to discuss in subsequent chapters views on the interrelations of carbohydrate and amino acid metabolism which by their molecular structure can influence the metabolism of nervous tissue at the level of glycolysis as well as at the level of the tricarboxylic acid cycle.

FORMATION OF LACTIC ACID IN RELATION TO NEURONAL ACTIVITY AND DIFFERENT TYPES OF CORTICAL CELLS

During glycolysis energy is obtained by reactions where inorganic phosphate is bound with monosaccharides to phosphate esters with a low energy content; the latter are in a system of consecutive enzyme reactions transferred to 3-carbon phosphate compounds with a high energy content which is transmitted to the adenyl system. The intensity of glycolysis is conditioned by the ratio of $ADP + P_i/ATP$ and by the concentration of different products of anoxidative and oxidative metabolism in tissues; the ATP level and formation of energy rich $\sim P$ in the mitochondrial system of electron transport are considered the main control mechanisms as regards the intensity of glycolysis (Lardy and Parks 1956, Passonneau and Lowry 1962, Sacktor 1966) because they limit the activity of hexokinase and phosphofructokinase resp., similarly as the concentration of different products of the anoxidative and oxidative metabolism (Garland, Randle and Manchester 1962, Garland, Randle and Newsholme 1963, Hess 1963).

The rise in neuronal activity *in vitro* or *in situ* is associated with a rise in lactic acid in tissue (e. g. Dixon 1949, McIlwain 1959, Bain and Pollock 1949, Klein and Olsen 1947, Richter and Dawson 1948, Gerard 1955, Ruščák 1962 and others). So far we do not possess reliable data on the cell elements which condition the formation and rise of lactic acid in nervous tissue during its excitation. From the work of Friede (1965) and Rose (1967) it may be concluded that lactic acid is formed mainly in the glia, as the latter has a much higher lactate dehydrogenase activity than neurons. If we consider, however, on the other hand the fact that the carrier of functions in nervous tissue is not the glia but the neuron, we must investigate to what extent the formation of lactic acid is influenced by neurons, in particular during stimulation of nervous tissue. This problem was studied by comparing the lactic acid formation *in vitro* and *in situ* in the intact cortex and in the cortex with a decreased nerve cell number as described in previous chapters.

The slices were incubated for 1 hr in an atmosphere of O_2 in Warburg vessels at 37 °C with 6.6 mM glucose and after deproteinization of the tissue together with the medium with 1 N $HClO_4$

Table 14

	I		II	
	C	E	C	E
a	585 ± 27	675 ± 30	107 ± 5	144 ± 10
	$P < 0.05$		$P < 0.01$	
b	1965 ± 110	1625 ± 90	420 ± 13	349 ± 16
	$P < 0.05$		$P < 0.01$	

Lactic acid in μmoles as M ± S. E. M./g N_2 in the rat brain cortex incubated *in vitro* (I) in the Krebs-Ringer phosphate solution with 6.6 mM glucose as the substrate in the presence of 5 (a) or 105 (b) mM KCl and *in situ* (II) in non-stimualted state (a) or after Pentazol stimulation (b). C — intact cortex, E — cortex with relative predominance of non-neuronal elements. Mean values of 10 experiments.

61

the produced lactic acid was determined. In another series of experiments the heads of undecapitated animals were fixed with liquid air in the non-stimulated state as well as after Pentazole stimulation 90 sec after the onset of seizures and the isolated cortex was taken for lactate estimations.

The results summarized in table 14 show that in the non-stimulated tissue *in vitro* as well as *in situ* always higher values of lactic acid in the cortex with a relative predominance of non-nerve cells were found. When, however, the tissue was stimulated either *in vitro* by increasing the level of external potassium to 105 mM or *in situ* by i. p. Pentazole administration, always more lactic acid was found in the intact cortex. The rise in lactate after stimulation is even more marked when the absolute differences before and after stimulation of control cortex and cortex with a reduced number of nerve cells are compared. Thus *in vitro* in the intact cortex after potassium stimulation lactic acid rose on an average by 1380 μmoles/g N_2/hr, while in slices with a predominance of glia only by 950 μmoles/g N_2/hr. A similar picture was obtained in experiments *in situ* when after Pentazole stimulation lactic acid in the intact cortex rose by 313 μmoles/g N_2, while in the cortex with a reduced number of nerve cells it rose only by 205 μmoles/g N_2. The activity of lactate dehydrogenase estimated spectrophotometrically according to Kornberg (1955) was in the cortex with a predominance of glia only insignificantly higher: 2.7 μmoles/min/mg protein in the control and 2.95 μmoles/min/mg protein in the experimental cortex.

Also stimulation of the metabolism by ouabain or omission of calcium from the incubation medium was associated with a higher formation of lactic acid in the intact cortex. When slices of the cerebral cortex of rats with an intact and reduced number of nerve cells in a medium with ouabain were incubated, less lactic acid was found in the slices with a reduced number of nerve cells (1000 $\pm$ 30 as compared with 1200 $\pm$ $\pm$ 60 μmoles/g N_2 after 1 hr incubation; $n = 9$, $P < 0.02$). By omitting Ca^{++} from the medium the lactic acid formation was also lower in the slices with a relative predominance of non-neuronal elements (1600 $\pm$ 45 μmoles/g N_2 in slices of the experimental cortex and 1900 $\pm$ 80 μmoles/g N_2 in the control cortex; $n = 8$, $P < 0.02$).

From the presented results it is obvious that the formation of lactic acid in cerebral cortex is not simply a matter of the glia despite its high lactate dehydrogenase activity. It is possible that the glia breaks down glucose evenly to 3-carbon compounds and that due to the reduction of nerve cells the latter cannot be further used in oxidative processes which are limited by neurons (Rose 1967); therefore, due to the low oxidative metabolism of the glia they are to a greater extent reduced to lactate. On the other hand, during stimulation of the cortical metabolism *in vitro* as well as *in situ* the increased production of lactic acid depended primarily on nerve cells. Because the lactate dehydrogenase activity of the glia is higher than that of the nerve cells (Rose 1967), we assume that during stimulation of the cortex lactic acid is formed in the glia, however, as a result of stimuli which originate in the nerve cells, as the glia alone does not respond to stimulation by increased lactate formation.

FORMATION OF LACTIC ACID IN ISOLATED SUBCELLULAR STRUCTURES OF CEREBRAL HEMISPHERES IN RATS

A) PREPARATION OF SUBCELLULAR FRACTIONS

The method for preparation of subcellular fractions from brain was described by Brody and Bain (1952). Based on the experience with fractionation of other tissues, in particular the liver, they elaborated two procedures for the preparation of nuclear, mitochondrial, microsomal and soluble fractions. They homogenized the tissue in sucrose, centrifuged it at 800, 1500, 12,000 and 23,000 g and thus they obtained four fractions: nuclear, mitochondrial, microsomal and soluble. As it was, however, revealed later the method of isolation of subcellular fractions from the CNS was much more complicated than from parenchymatous organs such as liver or kidney. For example, in the liver the cell nuclei of the parenchyma account for ca 3/4 of the total number of nuclei of the organ; whereas, in the hemispheres the nuclei of the nerve cells, i. e. the functional elements of the CNS, account only for ca 20 % (Nurnberger 1958, Waelsch 1959). The heterogeneity of the material as regards shape, embryonic origin and function makes us also assume that the material obtained by fractionation will not be homogeneous as regards metabolic function and morphology. The first investigation of the fraction described as mitochondria confirmed this assumption. Whittaker (1959) and Whittaker and Gray (1962) investigated the composition of the mitochondrial fraction obtained from the hemispheres under the electron microscope and found that this fraction contained much more non-mitochondrial structures than mitochondria. Therefore they centrifuged this mitochondrial fraction against a discontinuous sucrose density gradient; in this way they obtained from the original mitochondrial fraction three sub-fractions which differed morphologically as well as by the distribution of enzymes involved in the synthesis and breakdown of acetylcholine. Thus at the boundary between 0.25 M and 0.8 M sucrose they obtained the lightest sub-fraction containing mainly fragments of myelin and membranes. At the boundary between 0.8 M and 1.2 M sucrose they found material which reminded by its appearance under the electron microscope of nerve endings filled with synaptic vesicules and partly with preserved synapses, i. e. with pre- and postsynaptic structures. This fraction contained mainly the enzymes acetylcholine-esterase and-or-synthetase. The third sub-fraction sedimenting in 1.2 M sucrose contained swollen mitochondria and also the main portion of succinate dehydrogenase activity was bound to it. A similar procedure was also used subsequently by other authors when separating the mitochondrial fraction. They divided it into a greater number of sub-fractions according to the sedimentation in media of different density (de Robertis et al. 1962) and instead of sucrose they used sucrose mixed with Ficoll (Tanaka and Abood 1963). (The technique and evaluation of results of fractionation of the CNS are discussed in greater detail in a review by Whittaker 1965.)

Our procedure of fractionation of the hemispheres with regards to available equipment was as follows: after removal of the bases and the rhomboencephalon the hemispheres were homogenized in a plexiglass homogenizer with a 90-μ slit between the wall and piston in 0.25 M sucrose. The nuclear fraction was removed from the homogenate at 900 g. The sediment was rehomogenized and centrifuged at the same rate for 10 min. The crude mitochondrial fraction was obtained from the supernatant fluid by centrifuging at 12,000 g for 30 min. Part of this fraction was used for experiments and the remainder after rehomogenizing in 0.25 M sucrose was placed on a prepared sucrose gradient of 0.8, 1.0 and 1.2 M and centrifuged at 30,000–50,000 g for 60 min. The separated four sub-fractions were sucked off, diluted at a ratio of 1:1 with a medium without substrate and centrifuged again for 20 min. The supernatant after removal of the crude mitochondrial fraction was centrifuged at 30,000 g for 60 min. Thus we obtained the membrane fraction and a supernatant which did not sediment at this centrifugal force. The separation was made on a centrifuge MSE 17 angle head 69 181 at — 2 °C and the last experiments were carried out on an ultracentrifuge VAC 60, Rotor N^r 3208. From the crude mitochondrial fraction, as well as the sub-fractions obtained by separation on a sucrose density gradient, ultrathin sections were prepared for observation under the electron microscope: the common procedure of fixation with 1 % buffered osmic acid, pH 8.6, in 0.25 M sucrose, and embedding in an Epon mixture was used. The ultrathin sections were photographep under an electron microscope JEM 7.

The electronmicroscopic examinations revealed that in the crude mitochondrial fraction (CM) there were in addition to mitochondria also myelin fragments and fragments of nerve cell processes as well as nerve endings (fig. 12). The separation of the mitochondrial fraction into four sub-fractions against a sucrose density gradient rendered it possible to separate roughly the myelin (I), membranes and light nerve endings (II), heavy nerve endings (III) and mitochondria (IV). The sub-fraction sedimenting at the boundary of 0.25 M and 0.8 M sucrose contained mainly myelin fragments with occasional fragments of synaptic endings and small mitochondria (fig. 13). In the sub-fraction at the boundary of 0.8 M and 1.0 M sucrose different structures were found: among them fragments of myelin, membranes and nerve endings with some mitochondria predominated (fig. 14). The sub-fraction obtained between 1.0 M and 1.2 M sucrose contained mainly nerve endings with mitochondria (fig. 15). The last fraction sedimenting in 1.2 M sucrose contained swollen mitochondria, occasional nerve endings and lysosomal structures (fig. 16). The fraction described as membrane fraction, sedimenting at 30,000 g, contained membraneous structures and some mitochondrial fragments, nerve endings and ribonucleoprotein particles (fig. 17). In order to obtain a purer membrane fraction we used in the primary fraction an osmotic disruption in distilled water. By repeated centrifuging after osmotic disruption the vesicular structures were removed and as will be demonstrated, its enzymatic properties were also changed.

As regards the distribution of nitrogen insoluble in 1 N HClO$_4$ we found the following distribution in the hemispheres: homogenates of hemispheres with a mean weight of 1.50 g had on an average 29.1 mg N$_2$; 6.84 mg (23.5 %) was found in the crude mitochondrial fraction, 8.05 mg (27.6 %) in the membranes and supernatant and the remainder was in the fraction sedimenting at 900 g. Individual sub-fractions

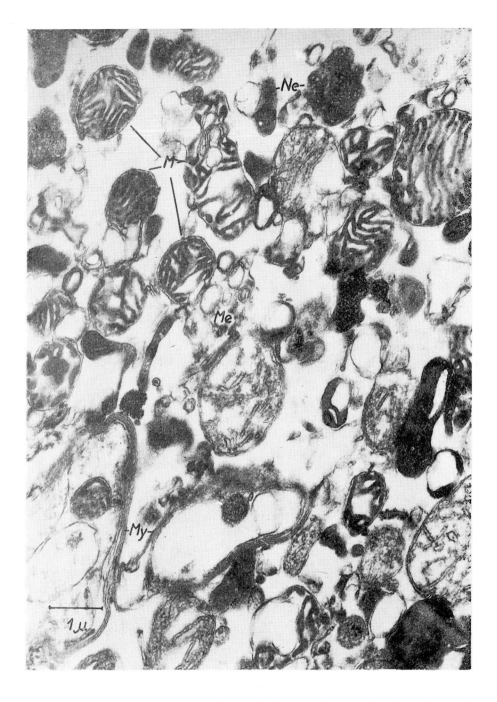

Fig. 12. Electronmicrograph of the crude mitochondrial fraction. My — myelin, M — mitochondria, Me — membranes, Ne — nerve endings.

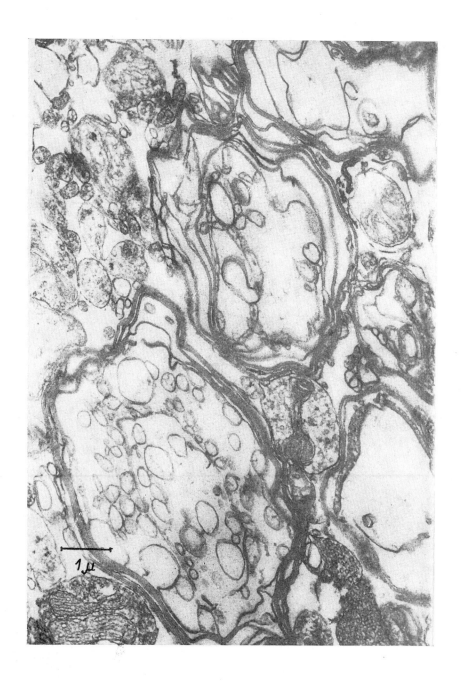

Fig. 13. Electronmicrograph of the material obtained at the borderline between 0.25 and 0.8 M sucrose. Its main component was myelin.

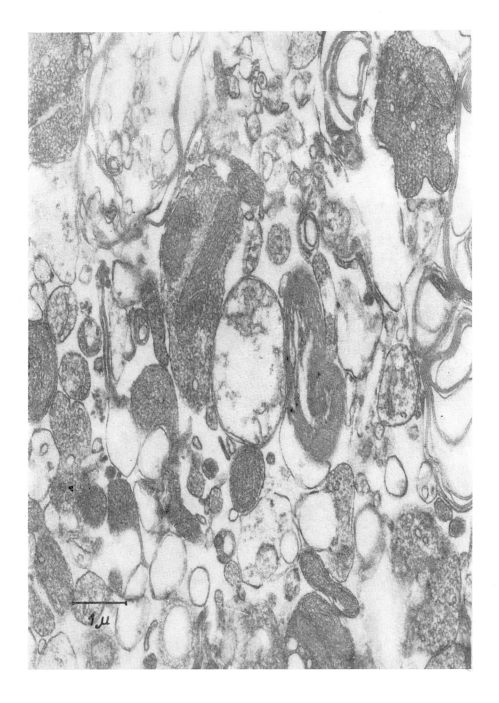

Fig. 14. Electronmicrograph of the sub-fraction sedimented between 0.8 and 1 M sucrose containing predominantly fragments of nerve endings and membranes.

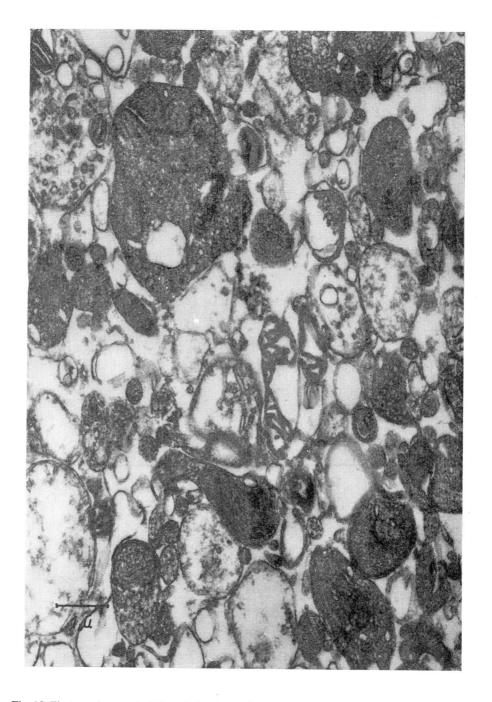

Fig. 15. Electronmicrograph of the sub-fraction sedimented between 1 and 1.2 M sucrose consisting mainly of nerve endings.

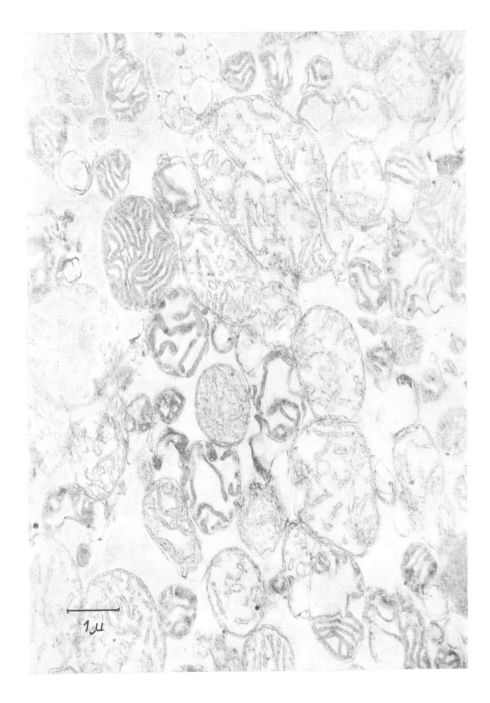

Fig. 16. Electronmicrograph of a fraction sedimented in 1.2 M sucrose. Swollen mitochondria were its main component.

71

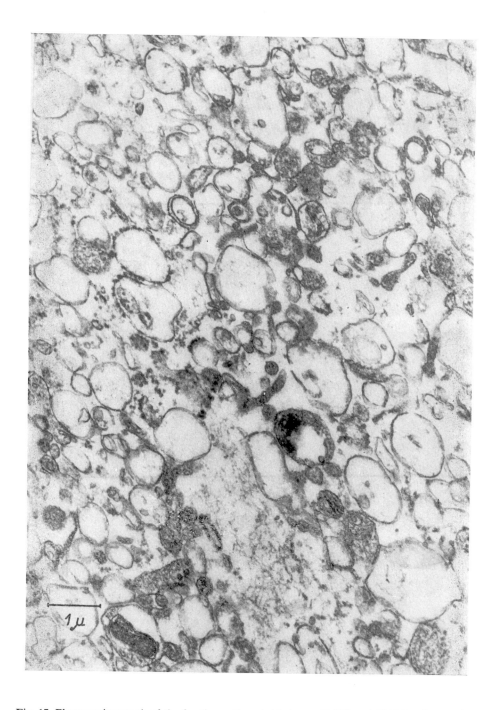

Fig. 17. Electronmicrograph of the fraction sedimented between 12,000 and 30,000 g. It contained fragments of the membranous structures and nerve endings.

of the crude mitochondrial fraction, the values of which were taken as 100 %, had the following distribution: in the first sub-fraction there were 19.88 %, in the second 29.24 %, in the third 25.58 % and in the fourth 13.62 % of the total nitrogen. The difference of 11.68 % between the sum of nitrogen in individual sub-fractions and the crude mitochondrial fraction was probably due to the fact that it was not possible to analyze the entire material, as we wanted to avoid the mutual mixing of fractions when sucking them off.

As evident from our results, we were able to prepare from brain homogenates sub-fractions characterized by a predominance of a certain distinct morphological component in each one of them. Our data are almost identical with the findings of de Robertis et al. (1962) as far as the morphological appearance of individual sub-fractions is concerned as well as regards the distribution of nitrogen. We, too, observed in our experiments that sucrose caused, contrary to the findings with Ficoll (Tanaka and Abood 1963),[1] swelling of the mitochondria. As can be seen from experiments with the respiratory activity (described below), we were unable to prepare a pure sub-fraction. Each[1] one of them was to some extent contaminated — in particular by mitochondria and fragments of synaptic endings. These findings are in keeping with those of Tanaka and Abood (1963), who have reported a high incidence of mitochondria in the sub-fraction of nerve endings. The so-called membrane fraction contained, similarly as mentioned by Petrushka and Guiditta (1959), as its main component membrane fragments of uncertain origin, probably from cell processes and fragments of the endoplasmic reticulum with some fragments of nerve endings and ribonucleoprotein particles. This fraction contained under our experimental conditions also mitochondrial fragments and their respiratory activity was about 8 % of the values of the crude mitochondrial fraction.

B) FORMATION OF LACTIC ACID IN SUBCELLULAR STRUCTURES AND ITS RELATIONSHIP TO THE SUBSTRATE USED AND THE IONIC COMPOSITION OF THE MEDIUM

As mentioned above, we wanted to elucidate the localization of glycolytic processes taking place in substructures of the CNS. We considered this problem of particular interest because since the initial work of Brody and Bain (1952) ample material has been assembled on this problem, as regards the volume of publications and controversial character of views. Brody and Bain (1952) have maintained that glycolysis in the CNS is not bound to the mitochondrial but to the soluble cytoplasmic fraction. Their views are also shared by Johnsson (1960) and Beattie, Sloan and Basford (1962). Some authors maintain that the mitochondrial fraction contains a substantial part of hexokinase of the CNS (Basford et al. 1964, Bachelard 1966) and that the latter, contrary to hexokinase soluble in cytoplasm, which is responsible for basic glycolysis in nervous tissue, is involved in metabolic processes under conditions of enhanced energy production (Johnsson 1960). This view is also supported by the experiments of Cremer (1960) who found that when mitochondria were added to the supernatant obtained from the hemispheres, the lactate production increased markedly. From these and other similar results (Beattie, Sloan and Basford 1962, Schwarz and Lee Kwang Loo 1960) the conclusion is drawn that mitochondria of the brain can influence by their hexokinase content the intensity of glycolysis in the intact nervous tissue as a whole.

There are, however, also data on the glycolytic ability of mitochondria isolated from the CNS. Hesselbach and du Buy (1953) prepared the mitochondrial fraction from a sucrose homogenate, incubated it under aerobic conditions with glucose as substrate and found that the mitochondrial fraction consumed under these conditions O_2 (they did not record, however, O_2 consumption by the supernatant); at the same time lactate was produced from glucose, about one third in relation to the amount of lactate produced by the supernatant. Gallagher, Judah and Rees (1956) found that lactate was formed from glucose in mitochondria prepared from 0.25 M sucrose and that it was further oxidized in the tricarboxylic acid cycle as suggested by the presence of α-oxoglutarate in the incubation system. Balázs (1959) and Balázs and Lagnado (1959) reported that ca 10 % of the total glycolytic activity of the CNS was bound to mitochondria, and the remainder to the soluble cytoplasmic fraction. Mitochondria prepared in their experiments essentially by Brody and Bain's method (1952) were able to break down glucose to lactate and to utilize it further in the oxidative cycle. They found a relative increase of lactate in the mitochondrial fraction under anaerobic conditions in an atmosphere of N_2. When the mitochondrial fraction was rinsed with physiological saline, the glycolysis in this fraction declined also. Among the tested enzymes of the glycolytic cycle in the mitochondrial fraction triosephosphate dehydrogenase had the lowest activity and from this finding the conclusion was drawn that the triosephosphate dehydrogenase activity is the limiting factor which determines the intensity of glycolysis in mitochondria.

Abood, Brunngraber and Taylor (1959) found almost one third of the total glycolytic activity of the CNS in the mitochondrial fraction and confirmed that in the cerebral mitochondria, contrary to those in the liver, heart and kidney, enzymes were present which could utilize glucose by the glycolytic and subsequently the oxidative pathway. Two of the above quoted authors found later (Brunngraber and Abood 1960) that the mitochondrial fraction produced lactate in equal amounts from glucose and fructose-1,6-diphosphate, whereby hexokinase stimulated only the production of lactate from glucose but not from fructose-1,6-diphosphate; they also claim, in keeping with the assumption of Balázs and Lagnado (1959), that in addition to hexokinase there is another enzyme, somewhere after the hexose diphosphate step, limiting glycolysis in the mitochondrial fraction. The addition of glyceraldehyde-3-phosphate dehydrogenase, aldolase and lactate dehydrogenase resp., did not influence, however,

74

the intensity of glycolysis in the mitochondrial fraction. Cohen (1961) found that mitochondria of the CNS could utilize by the glycolytic way glucose as well as fructose, glucose-6-phosphate as well as fructose-1,6-diphosphate. It was assumed that mitochondria of the brain differ as to their glycolytic properties substantially from mitochondria of other organs. Glycolysis in the cerebral mitochondria was assumed to be the factor which promptly renders possible an increased energy production which is frequently required by nerve cells to cope with their functional load. This is accomplished in such a way that at the very site of oxidative processes in mitochondria substrates are formed which are utilized in processes of oxidative phosphorylation (Gallagher Judah and Rees 1956, du Buy and Hesselbach 1956).

Subsequently, however, papers were published suggesting that mitochondria of the brain did not differ as regards their glycolytic properties from mitochondria of the heart, liver and kidneys resp. and that the glycolytic properties of mitochondria isolated from the brain are not bound to the latter but to other components which are formed during the blending of nervous tissue and which sediment at the same centrifugal forces as mitochondria (Aldridge 1957, Brunngraber, Aguilar and Occomy 1963). Direct evidence of the absence of glycolysis in brain mitochondria was produced by the work of Tanaka and Abood (1963) as well as our own work (Ruščák, Macejová and Ruščáková 1964 and Ruščák et al. 1964). Tanaka and Abood (1963) centrifuged the mitochondrial fraction obtained in the usual way against a discontinuous density gradient with Ficoll and separated it into four sub-fractions: in the lightest one they detected in the electron microscope fragments of white matter and axons, in the next one synaptic endings, then synaptic endings mixed with mitochondria and in the last one mainly mitochondria. Investigating the lactate production in these four sub-fractions, they found the highest glycolysis in the first and second sub-fraction, while in the fourth — mitochondrial one — they found only 0.8% of the total glycolytic activity of the crude mitochondrial fraction.

As the views on glycolysis in different subcellular structures isolated from the CNS have been very controversial, we shall now submit our views and results of our own experiments.

Fractions obtained by the procedure described in the preceding chapter were incubated in a medium with the following final composition: NaCl 100 mM, KCl 10 mM, potassium-phosphate buffer 20 mM, $MgCl_2$ 5 mM, ATP 2 mM, NAD 0.2 mM and substrates as listed in the tables. The incubation took place in 4 ml medium in Warburg manometric flasks for 1 hr at 37 °C in an atmosphere of air. After 1 hr the incubated preparations were deproteinized with 1 ml 20 % trichloracetic acid or 1 ml 2.5 N $HClO_4$ resp., and in the supernatant lactic acid using Barker-Summerson's method (1941), was estimated; the determined results are given as the arithmetic mean $\pm$ S. E. M. in μmoles per g N_2 insoluble in the deproteinizing agents. The N_2 was determined after mineralization of the sediment with H_2SO_4 by distillation of the produced ammonia. The results were evaluated statistically by the t-test.

Table 15

	Glc	Glc + Glu	Glc + GABA	Glc-1-P	Glc-1-P + Glu	Glc-1-P + GABA	Fru-1,6-diP	Fru-1,6-diP + Glu	Fru-1,6-diP + GABA
Phosphate buffer	2066 ± 57	2045 ± 29	2010 ± 77	484 ± 51	476 ± 20	450 ± 12	2358 ± 25	1613 ± 160	1630 ± 108
Tris buffer	3000 ± 44	—	—	881 ± 45	—	—	2461 ± 170	—	—

Lactic acid in μmoles as M ± S. E. M./g N_2 produced after 2 hr incubation of the crude mitochondrial fraction in Krebs-Ringer phosphate solution in the air atmosphere with the following substrates: 6.6 mM glucose (Glc), 6.6 mM glucose + 7 mM L-glutamic acid (Glc + Glu), 6.6 mM glucose + 10 mM GABA (Glc + GABA), 6.6 mM glucose-1-phosphate (Glc-1-P), 6.6 mM glucose-1-phosphate + 7 mM L-glutamic acid (Glc-1-P + Glu), 6.6 mM glucose-1-phosphate + 10 mM GABA (Glc-1-P + GABA), 6.6 mM fructose-1,6-diphosphate (Fru-1,6-diP), 6.6 mM fructose-1,6-diphosphate + 7 mM L-glutamic acid (Fru-1,6-diP + Glu), 6.6 mM fructose-1,6-diphosphate + 10 mM GABA (Fru-1,6-diP + GABA). Mean values of 10 experiments.

From table 15 it is evident that the crude mitochondria broke down glucose to lactate. Lactate was also form d when glucose-1-phosphate or fructose-1,6-diphosphate was used as subs rate, the formation of lactic acid being lowest with glucose-1-phosphate. Our experiments with the addition of L-glutamate or GABA to the above substrates were stimulated by the results of experiments with brain cortex slices where the use of both substrates led to a significant increase in lactate formation (table 16). Neither L-glutamate nor GABA had any effect on the lactate production in crude mitochondria. When Tris instead of phosphate buffer under the same experimental conditions was used, the lactate formation increased, but even then the lactate formation was lowest with glucose-1-phosphate.

As the electron microscopic investigations showed that the crude mitochondrial fraction contained also nonmitochondrial structures, to which the glycolytic activity could be bound, in subsequent work we focussed our attention on obtaining more homogeneous preparations. After separating the crude mitochondrial fraction against a sucrose density gradient into four sub-fractions it was found that the lactate production from glucose in these sub-fractions different significantly (table 17). In sub-fraction I at the boundary 0.25 − 0.8 M sucrose after 1 hr incubation 907 μmoles lactate/g N_2 were found; in sub-fraction II between 0.8 and 1.0 M sucrose 1443 μmoles lactate/g N_2; in sub-fraction III between 1.0 and 1.2 M sucrose the lactate content was highest − 1776 μmoles/g N_2, while

Table 16

	Glc	Glc + Glu	Glc + GABA
Phosphate buffer	2572 ± 100	4655 ± 330	3466 ± 85
Tris buffer	3500 ± 88	5237 ± 111	3244 ± 39

Lactic acid in μmoles as M±S. E. M./g N_2 in the rat brain cortex slices incubated 1 hr in the air atmosphere with the substrates : glucose (Glc), glucose + L-glutamic acid (Glc + Glu) and glucose + GABA (Glc + GABA). Concentrations of the substrates the same as in table 15. Mean values of 10 experiments.

Table 17

H	CM	M_1	M_2	M_3	M_4	Me	S
874 ± 109	1026 ± 78	907 ± 103	1443 ± 145	1776 ± 193	88 ± 21	273 ± 7	1026 ± 55

Lactic acid in μmoles as M ± S. E. M./g N_2 in the rat brain homogenates (H), crude mitochondrial fraction (CM) and its four sub-fractions (M_1, M_2, M_3, M_4), in the fraction of the membranes (Me) and in the supernatant (S) after 1 hr incubation of these subcellular fractions in Krebs-Ringer phosphate medium pH 7.4, in the air atmosphere with 6.6 mM glucose as the substrate. Mean values of 12 experiments.

in sub-fraction IV sedimenting in 1.2 M sucrose the amount of produced lactic acid was, as compared with the previous sub-fractions, only slight—88 μmoles/g N_2.

The difference between sub-fraction II and III is not statistically significant. There is, however, a statistically significant difference between the crude mitochondrial fraction and sub-fractions II and III and between sub-fraction I as compared with sub-fractions II and III. When we took the formation of lactate in the crude mitochondrial fraction as 100 %, then its formation in different sub-fractions was as follows: sub-fraction I—88.3 %, II—140.6 %, III—173.1 % and IV—8.5 %.

Next we compared the glycolysis of the total homogenates, of the mitochondrial fraction and the fraction not sedimenting at 12,000 g. If we take into account that of the total N_2 content 48.9 % were in the nuclear fraction, 23.5% in the mitochondrial fraction and 27.6 % in the supernatant, then, assuming that in the nuclear fraction glycolysis cannot take place, we reach the conclusion that the whole homogenate should produce under our experimental conditions on an average 821 μmoles lactate/g N_2. The actual production of 874 μmoles/g N_2 corresponds to the theoretically calculated value and is within the range of recorded results. These calculations confirm also that in the crude mitochondrial fraction glycolysis takes place. Glycolysis in the membrane fraction was, as compared with the crude mitochondrial fraction, relatively low, on an average 273 μmoles/g of insoluble nitrogen per hour.

The question therefore arose as to what extent the lactate production in the crude mitochondrial fraction was associated with the structures it contained or whether this process depended on the presence of enzymes of the glycolytic cycle

Table 18

	M	M_2	M_3
I	1026 ± 78	1443 ± 145	1776 ± 193
II	282 ± 15	642 ± 11	852 ± 8
III	208 ± 22	116 ± 29	870 ± 36

Lactic acid in μmoles as M $\pm$ S. E. M./g N_2 in the crude mitochondrial fraction (M) and its M_2 and M_3 sub-fractions isolated from rat brain hemispheres after 1 hr incubation in Krebs-Ringer phosphate solution with 6.6 mM glucose as the subtrate in the air atmosphere without osmotic shock (I) and after washing with distilled water once (II) on three times (III) respectively. Mean values of 10 experiments.

in cytoplasmic fragments present in this fraction. One of the possible procedures we used was rinsing the crude mitochondrial fraction with distilled water. We assumed that in this way we could cause an osmotic disruption of structures present in the mitochondrial fraction and thus release enzymes of the glycolytic cycle into water. In experiments where an osmotic disruption of the crude mitochondrial fraction was evoked (table 18) we found that after rinsing with distilled water the lactate formation decreased by 72.5 % as compared with experiments where a 0.9 % solution of NaCl was used for rinsing. While after rinsing with saline after 1 hr incubation in glucose we detected 1026 ± 78 μmoles lactate/g N_2, after rinsing with distilled water the lactate formation decreased to 282 ± 5 μmoles/g N_2. We assume that this result provides evidence that the enzymes of the glycolytic cycle are not bound to morphologically defined structures in the mitochondrial fraction but that they are present mainly as constituents of the cellular cytoplasm in structures covered by membranes such as nerve endings. In order to confirm this assumption we used for experiments the fraction of nerve endings after its osmotic disruption with distilled water. In these experiments, too, we found a similar reaction.

While in nerve endings rinsed with the incubation solution a lactate formation of 1776 μmoles/g N_2/hr was recorded, in the same fraction after rinsing with water instead of the incubation medium the lactate formation decreased to 852 μmoles/g N_2/hr. Also in sub-fraction II the lactate production after 1 hr incubation following rinsing with distilled water declined from 1443 to 642 μmoles/g of insoluble nitrogen. In order to assess whether the observed decline of lactate production will continue, in subsequent experiments we rinsed the membrane fraction and sub-fractions II and III of the crude mitochondrial fraction three times with distilled water. It was observed that in sub-fraction II the lactate production declined to 116 μmoles/g N_2, while in sub-fraction III it remained approximately at the same level of 870 μmoles/g N_2. In the membrane fraction lactate was not produced after rinsing. These experiments confirmed our view that the lactate production in morphologically defined subcellular structures is conditioned by the presence of cytoplasmic en-

Table 19

	Glc	Glc+Glu	Glc+GABA	Glc-1-P	Glc-1-P+Glu	Glc-1-P+GABA	Fru-1,6-diP	Fru-1,6-diP+Glu	Fru-1,6-diP+GABA
Phosphate buffer	2169 ± 51	2091 ± 56	2496 ± 52	1612 ± 52	1694 ± 104	1726 ± 56	1455 ± 78	1613 ± 140	1360 ± 33
Tris buffer	3391 ± 375	—	—	1872 ± 123	—	—	2107 ± 179	2047 ± 374	—

Oxygen consumption in μmoles as M ± S. E. M./g N_2 after 2 hr incubation of the crude mitochondrial fraction. Experimental conditions the same as reported in table 15.

zymes of the glycolytic cycle which are either adsorbed to these structures or are present in parts of cytoplasm contained in the different subcellular fractions.

Also sonic disruption and subsequent rinsing of the crude mitochondrial fraction with the incubation medium without substrate caused a significant decrease in lactate production, the amount of which declined in thus prepared fractions after 1 hr incubation to 586 ± 13.2 μmoles/g N_2 ($n = 6$). Similarly as after osmotic disruption, after the above procedure the glycolytic properties of the membrane fraction completely disappeared.

In addition to aerobic glycolysis we also investigated the O_2 consumption of the crude mitochondrial fraction and of individual sub-fractions. After 2-hr incubation of the crude mitochondrial fraction in Warburg manometric flasks at 37 °C in phosphate buffer with 2 mM ATP + 0.2 mM NAD, pH 7.4 with glucose, glucose-1-phosphate or fructose-1,6-diphosphate the O_2 consumption was recorded. The latter was not influenced, similarly as in the case of glycolysis, by addition of L-glutamate and GABA resp. to the mentioned substrates (table 19). Most intense respiration was recorded with glucose as substrate; when Tris buffer was added, this phenomenon was even more marked.

Similarly as in the crude mitochondria, also in the sub-fractions not only glycolysis took place but O_2 was also consumed (table 20). The O_2 consumption was highest in sub-fraction III where nerve endings with mitochondria predominated. The respiration of individual sub-fractions is due to their contamination with mitochondria or their fragments resp.: the lighter mitochondria and their fragments sediment together with the non-mitochondrial formations in sucrose of lower molarity and their enzymatic system is able to transport electrons and to

Table 20

M$_1$	M$_2$	M$_3$	M$_4$
250 ± 40	651 ± 21	823 ± 67	153 ± 25

Oxygen consumption in μmoles as M ± S. E. M./g N$_2$ in four sub-fractions isolated from crude mitochondrial fraction after 1 hr incubation in Krebs-Ringer phosphate medium with 6.6 mM glucose as the substrate. Mean values of 12 experiments.

utilize substrates which are formed during glycolysis by the oxidative cycle.

Glycolysis in nervous tissue is closely related to active ion transport across the membrane, as was previously demonstrated when we incubated cortical slices from rabbits in Krebs-Ringer solution under anaerobic conditions in an atmosphere of N$_2$: CO$_2$ = 95 : 5 in the presence of 20 μM ouabain. We found that ouabain inhibited anaerobic glycolysis by blocking the active ion transport across the membrane. Therefore in subsequent experiments we concentrated our attention on investigations of glycolysis in relation to the ionic composition of the medium and active transport. It was observed that glycolysis was more intense in the crude mitochondrial fraction and the membrane fraction when the medium contained Na$^+$ and K$^+$ ions. A similar effect as by the elimination of Na$^+$ ions was produced by ouabain in a concentration of 200 μM. Neither ouabain nor a pure potassium medium had any influence on the lactate production in the supernatant (for summarized results see table 21).

The results of our experiments are in keeping with data in the literature, i. e. that the crude mitochondrial fraction obtained by the method used for isolation of mitochondria from other organs was able to utilize glucose and to form lactic acid. At the same time we found that this fraction contained in addition to mitochondria

Table 21

	A	B	C
CM	888 ± 32 $n = 6$	626 ± 37 $P < 0.01$ $n = 6$	628 ± 77 $P < 0.01$ $n = 6$
Me	298 ± 10 $n = 6$	229 ± 4 $P < 0.01$ $n = 6$	243 ± 9 $P < 0.02$ $n = 6$
S	2302 ± 441 $n = 10$	2224 ± 45 $n = 10$	2221 ± 40 $n = 10$

Lactic acid in μmoles as M ± S. E. M./g N$_2$ produced after 1 hr incubation of the crude mitochondrial fraction (CM), membranes (Me) and supernatant (S) in the following media: A – NaCl 75 mM, KCl 55 mM, Tris pH 7.4 20 mM, MgCl$_2$ 3 mM, NAD 0.2 mM, ATP 1 mM, glucose 6.6 mM. B – A + 200 μM ouabain. C – NaCl replaced by KCl. Air atmosphere. n — number of experiments.

also non-mitochondrial particles as demonstrated e. g. by Petrushka and Guiditta (1959), de Robertis et al. (1962), Whittaker (1965) and others. Therefore we assumed that the glycolytic properties ascribed to mitochondria have not been experimentally confirmed and we investigated the glycolysis in individual sub-fractions obtained by centrifuging the crude mitochondrial fraction through a sucrose density gradient. Our findings, elaborated in detail, as well as those of Tanaka and Abood (1963) and Beattie, Sloan and Basford (1963) have shown that mitochondria devoid of non-mitochondrial sub-structures have practically no glycolytic properties and therefore do not differ from mitochondria of other organs, e. g. the liver and kidney (Aldridge 1957, Løvtrup and Zelander 1962), and that the enzymatic properties of the so-called crude mitochondrial fraction are not identical with the properties of mitochondria. Also de Robertis et al. (1962) and Whittaker (1959, 1965) provided evidence that pure mitochondria of the CNS differed as to their properties from the crude mitochondrial fraction; thus enzymes participating in the metabolism of acetylcholine are present only in synaptic endings and their fragments and not in mitochondria. On the other hand, Abood, Brunngraber and Taylor (1959) found that enzymes participating in oxidative phosphorylation are present only in mitochondria.

It is unlikely that the loss of glycolytic properties of pure mitochondria in our experiments was due to their swelling as their ATP-ase properties and their oxidative ability were also preserved under these conditions (Ruščák, Macejová and Ruščáková 1964, table 19 and 20).

After separation of the crude mitochondrial fraction into four sub-fractions we found that in sub-fraction II which contained membrane and nerve ending fragments and in sub-fraction III with nerve endings as much as 18 times more lactate was produced from glucose than in the pure mitochondrial fraction. In this respect our data differ from the results of Tanaka and Abood (1963) who found a maximum glycolysis in the so-called light fraction containing fragments of white matter and axons.

In order to find out whether the lactate production in the above fractions was bound to subcellular structures, we rinsed them with distilled water or disrupted them with ultrasound; we assumed that during osmotic or sonic disruption enzymes of the glycolytic cycle will be liberated into the water. A similar procedure for the detection of glycolytic enzymes in mitochondrial fractions was used also by Hesselbach and du Buy (1963) who found that hyposmotic disruption only reduced slightly the glycolytic activity of the mitochondrial fraction. Balázs and Lagnado (1959) after rinsing in Krebs-Ringer phosphate solution found, on the contrary, a reduction of the glycolytic activity of the crude mitochondrial fraction by as much as 50 %, but not so Brunngraber and Abood (1960) who after rinsing of the crude mitochondrial fraction with 0.25 M sucrose did not record any change in the glycolytic activity. We observed that the glycolysis practically disappeared in sub-fraction II but not in sub-fraction III even after rinsing three times with distilled water and these decrease by 45.4 % did not diminish after further treatment with distilled water. We assume therefore that glycolysis bound to nerve endings is conditioned by the presence of cytoplasmic inclusions in these formations which are resistant to hyposmosis. Glycolysis in the nerve endings could be directly associated with ensuring polarity of these structures by formation of energy in the anoxidative cycle. Evidence of the relationship between glycolysis and polarity of nervous tissue is provided also by our results, where we found on the one hand its stimulation in membranous and synaptic structures in a medium containing sodium and potassium and on the other hand a reduction of lactate formation in the same structures in the presence of ouabain. The formation of energy needed for preserving the polarity of nervous tissue can thus be regulated directly by the action of $Na^+ + K^+$-dependent ATP-ase by structures which regulate glycolysis by changes in the equilibrium of intracellular Na^+/K^+. The formed intermediary products of glycolysis can be further utilized in intramitochondrial oxidative processes of energy formation as the mitochondria responsible for the oxidative form of free energy production are in the close vicinity of membranes (Skou 1960) and synapses (Whittaker and Gray 1962).

The fact that in the third sub-fraction the highest glycolytic activity and O_2 consumption were found suggested that this fraction, as demonstrated also by electronmicroscopic observations, contained the greatest amount of cytoplasm and was strongly contaminated by mitochondria; thus the intermediary products of the glycolytic breakdown of glucose were in this sub-fraction further oxidized in the tricarboxylic acid cycle.

The relatively intense glycolysis in sub-fraction III also after rinsing with distilled water or after sonic disruption was a surprise to us. We are unable to differentiate whether the structures present in this sub-fraction are so resistant against ultrasound and hyposmosis that they are not completely disrupted or whether this fraction actually contains enzymes of the glycolytic cycle which are firmly bound to these structures. The disappearance of glycolytic properties after rinsing of the membranes rather suggests that the nerve endings, even after such drastic operations as those we used, preserved their structures partly intact; the latter contain permanently included parts of cytoplasm which is able to break down glucose to lactate.

When investigating the utilization of glucose and its phosphorylated derivatives we found that the basic substrate of glycolysis and respiration in the crude mitochondrial fraction was, in keeping with data reported in the literature (Brunngraber and Abood 1960, Cohen 1961), glucose and fructose-1,6-diphosphate and not glucose-1-phosphate. From this finding it may be concluded that the source of carbohydrates in the metabolism of nervous tissue is not glycogen but glucose and that the importance of glycogen for the metabolism of nervous tissue is slight as compared with muscle.

FREE AMINO ACIDS DURING DEPOLARIZATION OF THE CEREBRAL CORTEX IN SITU

The use of chromatographic methods rendered it possible to investigate amino acids in small specimens of material. Chromatography on paper and column chromatography revealed that in the mammalian brain there are almost all amino acids which enter peptide bonds, also in the so-called free, readily extractable form (Roberts, Frankel and Harman 1950, Tallan, Moore and Stein 1954). Glutamic and aspartic acid as well as their derivatives form with alanine almost 90 % of free amino acids; these amino acids are at the same time sites where the metabolic pathways of amino acids and those of keto acids, which form the carbon chain of the above amino acids (Braunstein 1949), may be mutually interconnected. Glutamic and aspartic acids and their derivatives as well as alanine having a common carbon chain with the keto acids involved in glycolysis and the tricarboxylic acid cycle were the subject of our further investigations, as they may possibly play a role as regulators of the tricarboxylic acid cycle and glycolysis (Braunstein 1947, 1957). At first we shall pay attention to the stationary levels of these amino acids in the cortex of rats and the results compare with those of other authors.

Amino acids were estimated in our material in ethanol extracts of cortical homogenates; the heads of the animals were fixed in liquid air and the cortex was removed by the method described in previous chapters. The amino acids were separated by means of paper chromatography in a solvent system n-butanol—acetic acid—water = 4 : 1 : 3, or by electrophoresis as described by Mikeš (1957) or by a combination of electrophoresis and chromatography. The paper was stained with a 0.5 % solution of ninhydrin in ethanol, the amino acid spots were fixed as described by Fischer — Dörfel (1953), eluated into methanol and readings of the color intensity were taken at 474 mμ. All values given in table 22 were calculated in μmoles and are given in μmoles per 100 g wet weight. The results proper were calculated per 100 g of brain from the results which are presented in the subsequent text in μmoles per gram of nitrogen insoluble in ethanol. The average nitrogen content in our experiments was 1.92 ± 0.04 g per 100 g wet weight of cortex.

If we compare the thus calculated results with those of other authors listed in table 22 they differ from some of the publications quoted. We recorded higher glutamine levels and a much lower concentration of GABA than reported by de Ruisseau et al. (1957) and Porcelatti and Thompson (1957), although their work on rat brains was made by paper chromatography and the tissue was also extracted by diluted ethanol. We assume that the different results are conditioned by a different procedure used for the preparation of the tissue extracts. While in our experiments the brains were first frozen in liquid air, and thus all enzymatic reactions were stopped, the above quoted authors froze the brains after removal from the skull or homogenized them without previous fixation in liquid air. This procedure can, however, lead to hydrolysis of glutamine and a rise in glutamic acid, as well as a rise in GABA which is known to increase in particular in conditions associated with brain anoxia (Elliot and van Gelder 1960, Gaevskaya and Nosova 1963). Comparison of values we recorded in rats with those found in other mammals have shown that there are practically no differences in the investigated amino acids among different species (Tallan, Moore and Stein 1954, Ginter 1958). Not even 30 min ligature of the carotids

Table 22

	Waelsch (1957)	Du Ruisseau et al. (1957)	Porcelatti and Thompson (1957)	Okumura et al. (+) (1959)	De Ropp and Snedeker (1960)	Herbert et al. (1966)	Own results carotids free	Own results carotids ligated
Asp	500	777	322	162	233	229	494	552
Glu	1000	1548	939	789	870	1020	844	785
GluNH$_2$	400	300	427	259	416	489	684	577
Ala	60	88	96	66	28	55	93	98
GABA	200	437	578	215	174	214	322	231

Some free extractable amino acids in the rat brain in μmoles/100 g wet wt according to the results of various authors. Paper chromatography or chromatography on column (+).

had any influence on the levels of the above-mentioned amino acids, except for a slight decrease in glutamic acid, this fact is in keeping with the findings of other authors (Thorn et al. 1958, Dravid and Jílek 1965) that during a reduced blood supply to the cerebral cortex its glutamic acid content is also lower. Our previous investigations concerning the content of glycogen, reducing substances, lactic acid, pyruvic acid, citric acid and α-oxoglutaric acid did not reveal any differences in the levels of these substances as compared with results in animals with an intact circulation and results obtained after 30-min ligature of the carotid arteries. Similarly histological examinations of the nervous elements (Ruščáková 1961, 1964) confirmed that 30-min ligature of the carotid arteries did not alter the histological appearance of nervous elements in the cerebral cortex. We must therefore assume that in anesthetized animals the metabolism of the cortex is maintained at such a level that even after ligature of the carotid arteries they meet the energy needs of the tissue without any influence on structures and functions; only during a concomitant functional load and a limited supply of substrate and O_2 by the blood does the brain use its own energy reserves, including amino acids, and make use of mechanisms which are to ensure under altered conditions energy for active nerve elements.

A) DICARBOXYLIC AMINO ACIDS AND DEPOLARIZATION OF THE CORTEX IN EEG DEPRESSION

Dicarboxylic amino acids are assumed to serve as a link between the metabolism of amino nitrogen and the tricarboxylic cycle as in the tricarboxylic cycle already complete carbon chains of dicarboxylic amino acids are formed, i. e. α-oxoglutaric and oxalacetic acids. Of these α-oxoglutaric acid can be transformed to glutamate by means of glutamic acid dehydrogenase which is found practically in all tissues (v. Euler, Adler, Günther and Das 1938). Glutamate dehydrogenase in the CNS is also, similarly as in other tissues, bound to the mitochondria (Brody and Bain 1952, Hogeboom and Schneider 1953, Klein 1956, Borst and Slater 1960). The highest activity of glutamic acid dehydrogenase in the CNS is in that part of the cerebral cortex which is concerned with motor function (Klein 1956). Its co-enzyme is pyridine nucleotide; it was found that it may be NAD and NADP, but NADP has only ca 10 % activity of NAD (Copenhaver, McShan and Meyer 1950, Schmidt 1956). The optimum pH for glutamic acid dehydrogenase is about 7.4 (Davis 1955, Schmidt 1956). The enzyme is strictly specific and is responsible for the reductive amination of α-oxoglutaric acid and the oxidative dehydrogenation of glutamic acid; the equilibrium in experiments *in vitro* is very much on the side of amination of α-oxoglutaric acid (Strecker 1957, Balázs 1965).

Glutamic acid may serve as a substrate of oxidation for nervous tissue. Krebs (1935) as well as Weil-Malherbe (1938, 1950) found that among different amino acids only glutamic acid was able to maintain the O_2 consumption of brain slices at the same level as glucose. On the other hand, the antimetabolite of glucose, 2-deoxyglucose causes *in vitro* a decrease in glutamic acid in brain slices (Tower 1960) whereby the O_2 consumption remains at the same level as during glucose utilization; this finding is also taken as evidence of the utilization of endogenous glutamic acid. The utilization by white matter is very low (Tower 1959). Mitochondria oxidize it much more than they decarboxylate it, which suggests that its oxidation follows predominantly a different route than that via the GABA shunt (Løvtrup 1961).

After glutamic acid administration into the circulation its level in the brain of adult animals does not change; therefore it was assumed that the barrier for it is impermeable (Waelsch 1951). Experiments with labelled ^{14}C glutamic acid revealed, however, that although the stationary level in the brain after systemic administration does not change, its exchange between blood and brain is more rapid (Lajtha, Berl and Waelsch 1959, Waelsch and Lajtha 1960, Roberts, Flexner and Flexner 1959). The high cerebral level suggests most probably that the main part of glutamic acid is formed directly in the brain by the above-mentioned reductive amination of α-oxoglutaric acid or in transamination reactions of α-oxoglutaric acid with other amino acids or by hydrolysis of glutamine (Weil-Malherbe 1950, McIlwain 1959).

Nervous tissue utilizes glutamic acid not only *in vitro* but also *in situ*. During insulin hypoglycemia the glutamic acid level declines, while the aspartic acid level rises. This is explained by the fact that during a reduced citric acid production, due to pyruvic acid deficiency, glutamic acid is transaminated with oxalacetic acid and the liberated α-oxoglutaric acid is further oxidized to oxalacetic acid which is able to bind further amino groups from glutamic acid (Dawson 1950, Tapia et al. 1967, de Ropp and Snedeker 1961, Massieu et al. 1962, Shaw and Heine 1965). A similar decrease in glutamic acid also occurs in the brain after administration of fluoroacetate (Dawson 1955). Fluoroacetate condenses with oxalacetic acid to fluorocitrate which inhibits aconitase activity (Peters 1955) and causes a decrease in isocitric and oxalsuccinic acids. In this case the brain utilizes glutamic acid, which, however, transaminates also with pyruvic acid which is formed during glycolysis when the condensation of pyruvic with oxalacetic to citric acid is reduced (Dawson 1955). The stimulation of the brain by electric current or drugs does not affect its level in the brain or causes only a slight decrease (Waelsch 1959).

Glutamic acid plays an important role in maintaining the potassium concentration of tissue. In a medium lacking glutamic acid potassium is lost from nervous tissue; when, however, glutamic acid is added, the accumulation of cellular K^+ returns also to normal values (Terner, Eggleston and Krebs 1950, McIlwain 1969). Its most important role is probably the regulation of the α-oxoglutaric and oxalacetic acid levels in the brain it acts as a buffer which controls the rate of the tricarboxylic acid cycle in the CNS (Swanson and Clark 1950, Waelsch 1957). It is assumed that the formation of α-oxoglutaric acid from glutamic acid in the brain takes place solely by transamination with α-keto acids (Strecker 1957, Krebs and Bellamy 1960, Balász 1965). Equally important is the function of glutamic acid as regards the incorporation of ammonia into amino acids and thus its inclusion into proteins.

Contrary to glutamic acid, after the parenteral administration of glutamine its level in the brain rises (Tigerman and McVicar 1961, Tower 1960); therefore it is assumed that glutamine is the transport form of glutamic acid and thus also of α-oxoglutaric acid to the brain. Glutamine is evenly distributed in the brain among all cell fractions and is found in an approximately equal concentration in gray and white matter (Palladin 1959); from this it is concluded that glutamine is not bound only to cell elements (Tower 1960). Its level in the brain is reduced during insulin hypoglycemia (Okumura, Otsuki and Nasu 1959). It has not been unequivocally resolved whether its first degradation product is glutamic acid or the amine of α-ketoglutaric acid, as it was revealed that in some tissues also transamination of keto acids with glutamine is possible (Meister 1956). Its drop during insulin hypoglycemia suggests that glutamine can be also used in the tricarboxylic acid cycle.

Aspartic acid cannot be formed by reductive amination from oxalacetate, as for a similar process so far the appropriate enzyme has not been found. Its function in the intermediary metabolism of the brain has not been elucidated in such detail as that of glutamic acid. In general it is maintained that dicarboxylic amino acids

88

as well as alanine have a key position in the regulation of the metabolism of the CNS because they are mutually linked by reversible transamination and cyclic interconversions with keto acids in the series of glycolysis and the tricarboxylic cycle (Braunstein 1957).

As apparent from the above brief review on the role of amino acids in the metabolism of nervous tissue the latter can influence its glycolytic as well as oxidative cycle. Therefore we focussed our subsequent experiments on investigations of amino acids which are closely related with glycolysis and the Krebs' cycle, in particular during prolonged depolarization of the cortex *in situ* which is associated with EEG depression during ligature of the carotid arteries. The first experiments showed that the EEG depression does not alter the stationary levels of aspartic and glutamic acid or of glutamine in the cortex with an intact circulation, even when for analyses only portions of the cortex in the negative phase of the EEG depression were used. When we applied, however, 3 M KCl for 30 min to the ischemic cortex after ligature of the carotid arteries, a significant decrease in aspartic and glutamic acid and glutamine in the cortex of the experimental hemispheres occurred, as can be seen from table 23.

Table 23

	I			II		
	C	E	n	C	E	n
GluNH$_2$	360 ± 13	330 ± 15	9	304 ± 6.5	235 ± 8	33
		n. s.			$P < 0.01$	
Glu	444 ± 16	420 ± 14	9	$361 \pm 10.$	289 ± 9.8	33
		n. s.			$P < 0.01$	
Asp	263 ± 19	256 ± 17	9	291 ± 13	238 ± 7	33
		n. s.			$P < 0.01$	

Glutamine (GluNH$_2$), glutamic acid (Glu) and aspartic acid (Asp) in μmoles as M $\pm$ S. E. M./g N$_2$ of control (C) and experimental (E) rat brain cortex following 30 min application of 3 M KCl to the cortex. I — carotid arteries free, II — carotid arteries ligated. Mean values of 9 (I) or 33 (II) experiments respectively. n. s. — differences statistically not significant.

B) RISE OF γ-AMINOBUTYRIC ACID IN THE CEREBRAL CORTEX DURING EEG DEPRESSION ELICITED AFTER LIGATURE OF THE CAROTID ARTERIES

Gamma-aminobutyric acid (GABA) was found in the brain of some mammals in 1950 by Roberts and Baxter and by Awapara et al. It was identified by Udenfriend (1950) by means of the isotope technique using ^{35}S and ^{131}I pipsyl GABA. Later it was detected in the brain of homoithermic as well as poikilothermic animals

(Roberts et al. 1958, Okumura, Otsuki and Nasu 1959, Frontali 1961) in approximately equal concentrations in different animal species. Although it is found in the nervous system in a readily extractable form in relatively high concentrations, it was not detected in brain proteins (Roberts 1960). It is bound to cell elements of the gray matter (Roberts and Baxter 1959, Albers and Brady 1959), to the mitochondrial fraction and the supernatant (Palladin 1959, Tower 1959).

GABA is formed by enzymatic decarboxylation of glutamic acid. The decarboxylation is probably an irreversible process, because fixation of $^{14}CO_2$ to GABA was not found (Roberts 1960). The enzyme was also found in nervous tissue of some invertebrates (Roberts et al. 1958, Frontali 1961). So far glutamic acid decarboxylase was not prepared in a crystalline form; however, some of its properties were already subjected to detailed investigations *in vitro* in experiments with brain homogenates. It was proved that the optimum pH for the activity of glutamic acid decarboxylase is ca 6.5; its activity rises during postnatal development and depends on vitamin B_6, which in phosphorylated form as pyridoxal-5-phosphate is a coenzyme of decarboxylase. The activity of glutamate decarboxylase is reduced by antimetabolites of vitamin B_6 (Roberts and Baxter 1960), KCN (Turský 1960) but not by anaerobic conditions. For the activity of the enzyme intact aldehyde group of coenzyme is essential as well as intact SH groups of the apoenzyme and Mn^{++} ions (Steensholt and Joner 1957, Roberts 1960).

It has not been decided unequivocally, however, to which cellular structures decarboxylase is bound. Some maintain that mitochondria are active (McKhann and Tower 1961, Shatunova and Sytinsky 1964), others proved that the decarboxylase activity was in the soluble cytoplasmatic fraction (Løvtrup 1961) and finally there is also evidence that it is present in specific nerve endings to which an inhibitory function in the CNS is ascribed (de Robertis 1967).

In vitro GABA is rapidly oxidized to succinic acid by brain slices as well as mitochondria (McKhann and Tower 1959, 1961). When GABA was used as the substrate for oxidation, the O_2 consumption was equally high as with other intermediary products of the tricarboxylic cycle. The oxidation rate increased in the presence of ADP; this proves that phosphate acceptors determine also the oxidation rate of GABA as a substrate (McKhann and Tower 1961). On the other hand, barbiturates and amytal inhibit its oxidation which suggests a connection between the intensity of GABA utilization and the system of electron transport across pyridine nucleotides (Sacktor, Cummins and Packer 1959).

GABA oxidation depends also on its ratio to other substrates in the incubation medium. When in the incubation medium the GABA concentration is high and the α-oxoglutaric acid content low, GABA is predominantly utilized. When, however, the α-oxoglutaric acid content is raised and that of GABA is reduced, oxoglutarate is utilized preferentially (McKhann and Tower 1961). For the further oxidation of GABA α-oxoglutaric acid is essential as from GABA its amino group to the latter is transferred and GABA is converted into succinic acid (Bessman, Rossen and Layne 1953, Roberts and Bregoff 1953, Baxter and Roberts 1958, Wilson, Hill and Koeppe 1959, Cacioppo, Pandolfo and di Chiara 1959).

The enzyme responsible for the transfer of the amino group from GABA to α-oxo-glutaric acid — GABA transaminase — is also found only in the gray matter of the brain (Salvador and Albers 1959) bound to mitochondria (Bessman, Rossen and Layne 1953). Its coenzyme is also pyridoxal-5-phosphate, the maximum activity is, however, at pH 8.2 and it is capable of transferring the amino group from GABA only to α-oxoglutaric acid which cannot be replaced in the transamination reaction by any other α-keto acid (Roberts and Baxter 1960). The bond of the coenzyme and apoenzyme is more labile in decarboxylase than in transaminase; therefore decar-boxylase is most sensitive to pyridoxal phosphate deficiency, *in vitro* as well as *in situ* (Tower 1958, Udenfriend, Weissbach and Mitoma 1960, Baxter and Roberts 1960). Transaminase is contained in mitochondria, as it was found that the activity of mitochondria was identical with the activity of whole brain homogenate (Baxter and Roberts 1960). The histochemical results of van Gelder (1965) revealed that trans-aminase activity is bound only to nerve elements and not to all types of cells present in the nervous tissue.

The intermediary product of GABA oxidation is supposed to be succinsemialde-hyde (Bessman, Rossen and Layne 1953, McKhann and Tower 1959, Albers 1960), for the latter in the brain a specific enzyme was found, which is able to oxidize synthetic succinsemialdehyde to succinate (Albers and Salvador 1958). The fact that succin-semialdehyde was not detected in the brain is explained by the high activity of its dehydrogenase which immediately transforms the produced succinsemialdehyde into succinate; that GABA is oxidized to succinate was confirmed by experiments with GABA $1-{}^{14}C$ where maximum activity was detected in succinic acid (Roberts, Rothstein and Baxter 1958).

In situ GABA is also formed from glutamic acid. When $U-{}^{14}C$ glutamic acid was administered to mice intracerebrally and the brains were analyzed $1-25$ mins after administration, already during the first minute GABA activity was detected (Roberts, Rothstein and Baxter 1958). Similarly Waelsch (1957) recorded a high GABA activity in mice following parenteral administration of $U-{}^{14}C$ glutamic acid.

The GABA level in brain is relatively stable and does not change even as a result of such processes as convulsions induced by electric stimuli or drugs (Roberts 1960). Its level is reduced after administration of convulsant hydrazides (Killam 1957, Baxter and Roberts 1959, Elliot and van Gelder 1960), antranyl-hydroxamic acid (Utley 1963), after antimetabolites of vitamin B_6 (Bukin 1959, Rindi and Ferrari 1959) and after reserpine (Balzer, Holtz and Palm 1961). Its rise was observed after administration of hydroxylamine which is supposed to inhibit the activity of GABA transaminase (Baxter and Roberts 1960), after administration of ethanol (Häkkinen and Kulonen 1959) aminooxyacetic acid (Wallach and Crittenden 1961) and during hypoxia (Elliot and van Gelder 1960, Maslova and Rozengart 1963). Woodbury and Vernadakis (1958) described a rise of GABA in the brain also after administration of diphenylhydantoin, acetazoleamide, adrenalin and after adrenalectomy; however, Roberts and Baxter (1960) considered this rise accidental.

The decrease of GABA in the brain after hydrazides, thiosemicarbazide or antimetabolites of vitamin B_6 is associated with an increased excitability of the CNS and convulsions which can be eliminated by the local application or subarachnoidal injections of GABA (Bukin 1957, Rindi and Ferrari 1959). On the other hand, an increase of GABA in the brain after injections of hydroxylamine should be associated with the decrease of excitability of the CNS (Eidelberg et al. 1959). Locally applied or intracerebrally injected GABA also reduces the spontaneous as well as evoked cortical activity (Grundfest 1958, Purpura et al. 1958, Jasper, Gonzales and Elliot 1958, Florey 1960, Honour and McLennan 1960) and therefore it has been assumed that GABA inhibits the synaptic transmission of impulses in the CNS and that the excitability of the CNS depends directly on the GABA level in the brain (Woodbury and Vernedakis 1958), whereby with the decrease of GABA the excitability should increase and *vice versa* (Woodbury and Epslin 1959, Udenfriend, Weissbach and Mitoma 1960). It is also admitted that the factor influencing the excitability of the CNS is not GABA itself but some of its derivatives found in the brain, such as γ-aminobutyrylcholine (Takahashi et al. 1959, McLennan 1958), or γ-guanidinebutyric acid which can be produced in the brain by transamidination of arginine with GABA (Ireverre et al. 1957, Blass 1960). Evidence of the inhibitory function of GABA is also provided by some work of de Robertis and his coworkers (de Robertis 1967, de Lores Arnaiz, Alberici and de Robertis 1967) who detected the presence of glutamate decarboxylase in the inhibitory nerve endings and therefore considered GABA the inhibitory transmitter in the CNS.

There are, however, also strong arguments against the inhibitory function of GABA in the brain. Thus it was found for instance that despite the absence of GABA in Factor I its inhibitory function was preserved (Honour and McLennan 1960), that GABA is found mainly in cell-bodies of neurons (Palladin 1959, Florey 1960), while processes and manifestations of excitability are predominantly synaptic phenomena. Moreover, it was observed that convulsive activity could be produced in an area of the brain with a high GABA content with smaller intensity of stimulation than in another area where the GABA content was lower (Baxter, Roberts and Eidelberg 1960). And, finally, a high and constant concentration of GABA in the brain would rather suggest the function of a regulator of the "milieu intérieur" in the brain than the function of a neurohormone (Baxter and Roberts 1960).

It is known that GABA stimulates the hexokinase activity in homogenates of the myocardium, skeletal muscle and to a certain extent also in brain homogenates (Bunyatyan 1963, Mori 1958); therefore GABA may also play a role in regulating the inten-

92

sity of the carbohydrate metabolism by exerting an influence on hexokinase. We cannot even rule out its function as a regulator of the tricarboxylic acid cycle in nervous tissue at the level of α-oxoglutaric acid—succinic acid via the "shunt" glutamic acid—GABA which can influence the energy metabolism of nerve elements and in this way probably also their function (Killam 1958, Sokoloff et al. 1959).

GABA can be also formed from glucose in the tricarboxylic acid cycle. This was demonstrated by experiments where brain slices were incubated in a medium with $U-{}^{14}C$ glucose (Beloff-Chain et al. 1955, Kini and Quastel 1959, Tsukada et al. 1960). It was also revealed that the GABA production in slices increased when the potassium concentration of the medium rose above the level of extracellular fluid. Potassium stimulated not only the GABA formation from glucose but also that of glutamine (Rybová 1960).

It is known from experiments (Křivánek and Bureš 1960, Brinley, Kandel and Marshall 1960) *in situ* that a temporary rise in extracellular potassium in nervous tissue occurs during the negative phase of the wave of spreading EEG depression. This temporary increase in extracellular potassium should also influence the GABA level during EEG depression. Moreover, the GABA level could increase as a result of a lower pH, caused by a rise in lactic acid which was observed during EEG depression, a higher activity of glutamic acid decarboxylase. And finally also temporary disappearance of electrical activity of the cortex during waves of depression, which could be associated with the rise of GABA, made us investigate in greater detail GABA in the brain of rats during EEG depression with a normal and reduced blood supply to the CNS.

It was demonstrated that the difference in GABA content between the right and left hemisphere of the same animal did not exceed the range of the method used (i. e. $\pm 8\%$). In seven animals with intact carotids we found in the cortex of one hemisphere 102 μmoles GABA/g N_2 and in the contralateral one 107 μmoles/g N_2. This finding made us use as control the intact cortex of the same animal. After 30 min local application of 3 M KCl to the cortex with intact circulation, which evokes repeated waves of spreading EEG depression and depolarization (Bureš and Burešová 1956) we did not record any significant increase in GABA in the cortex with EEG depression. In the control cortices we recorded GABA levels of 98 ± 5.7 μmoles/g N_2 and in the cortices with depression 106 ± 4 μmoles/g N_2. In subsequent experiments we investigated the GABA level only in that portion of the cortex which was in the phase of negativity. Under these experimental conditions we found a mild but insignificant rise in GABA in the depolarized area from an average of 101 ± 5 μmoles/g N_2 to 118 ± 9.8 μmoles/g N_2 ($n = 6$, $P < 0.2$).

In subsequent experiments KCl was applied to the cortex after bilateral ligature of the carotid arteries. It was found that 30 min ligature of the carotid arteries itself did not alter the GABA level of the brain, as compared with the results in experiments with intact circulation. The mean values of GABA after 30 min ligature of the carotid arteries were 104 ± 6 μmoles in one hemisphere and 108 ± 7.2 μmoles/g N_2 in the contralateral hemisphere of the same animal. GABA rose slightly already after 5 min action of 3 M KCl on the ischemic brain from an average level of 101 ± 8 μmoles/g N_2 to 117 ± 11 μmoles/g N_2. This rise proved to be insignificant ($P < 0.2$). However, the action of 3 M KCl on the ischemic brain led after 30 min to a significant rise in GABA in the cortex of the experimental hemispheres. From average values of $107 \pm 6 \mu$moles/g GABA rose to 186 ± 10 μmoles/g N_2 ($n = 40$, $P < 0.01$). The values of GABA in the control experiments did not differ from the controls observed in previous experiments after 30 min ligature of the carotid arteries. When the experimental hemisphere was divided into two portions, one of them exposed to the direct influence of KCl the other on which KCl did not act directly and over which only waves of negativity passed, in both portion an equal rise in GABA after 30 min action of 3 M KCl was found. From average values of 109 ± 6 μmoles/g N_2 GABA rose to 184 ± 7 μmoles/g N_2 in the area exposed to the direct action of KCl and to 195 ± 7.5 μmoles/g N_2 in those parts of the cortex over which only waves of negativity passed ($n = 20$, $P < 0.01$).

When 0.3 M KCl was applied, to the ischemic brain for 30 min, instead of 3 M KCl the GABA level rose in the experimental hemisphere from 104 ± 7 μmoles/g N_2 to 177 ± 9 μmoles/g N_2 ($n = 10$, $P < 0.01$).

If after 30 min action of 3 M KCl the trachea was compressed for 60 sec the GABA level in both hemispheres rose; however, the difference between the control and experimental cortex remained preserved. This rise in the GABA level reached 145 ± 17 μmoles/g N_2 in the control experiments and 263 ± 28 μmoles/g N_2 in the experimental hemispheres ($n = 10$, $P < 0.01$). Compression of the trachea for 150 sec abolished the differences between the experimental and control cortex because, as compared with the experiments without ligature of the trachea, the GABA level rose considerably in the control hemispheres. In the cortex exposed to the action of KCl the GABA level rose to 245 ± 30 μmoles/g N_2, and in controls it rose as high as 226 ± 21 μmoles/g N_2. As compared with the experimental cortex, there are no significant differences in the GABA content; however, the rise in GABA in the control cortex, as compared with the results of experiments without compression of the trachea, is statistically highly significant ($P < 0.01$).

We also investigated whether this rise in GABA after the action of KCl is a reversible process. It was observed that during ligature of the carotid arteries also after removal of KCl from the surface of the cortex the differences between the control and experimental hemispheres did not disappear. After 30 min restitution following 30 min action of 3 M KCl the same results were recorded as after 30 min exposure to KCl (120 ± 11 μmoles/g N_2 in the control and 208 ± 19 μmoles/g N_2 in the experimental cortices; $n = 10$, $P < 0.01$). Ninety minute restitution led to the elimination of differences in the GABA levels between control and experimental hemispheres because the GABA increase in the control hemisphere was greater than in the experimental one. Under these conditions the GABA level in the experimental hemispheres was 261 ± 32 μmoles/g N_2 and 251 ± 25 μmoles/g N_2 in the control

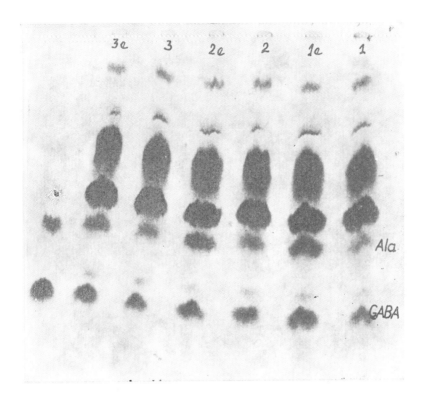

Fig. 18. Chromatogram of ethanol extracts of the control (1, 2, 3) and experimental (1e, 2e, 3e) rat brain cortex showing the rise in alanine (Ala) and GABA in the experimental cortex following 30 min KCl application after ligature of carotid arteries.

hemispheres ($n = 7$, $P < 0.5$). When the blood supply to the brain was renowed after 30 min action of KCl, after 30 min restitution the significant differences between control and experimental hemispheres already disappeared (120 ± 10 μmoles GABA/g N_2 in the controls and 149 ± 15 μmoles/g N_2 in the experimental hemispheres; $n = 9$, $P < 0.2$). The differences were even slighter after 90 min restitution; in control hemispheres GABA levels of 117 ± 8 μmoles/g N_2 were found and in experimental ones 128 ± 9 μmoles/g N_2 ($n = 10$, $P < 0.5$).

Since a similar metabolic effect as that produced by K^+ ions is also exerted by raised rubidium, cesium and ammonium ion concentrations in the medium (Dickens and Greville 1935, Weil-Malherbe 1956, Hertz and Schou 1962), in subsequent

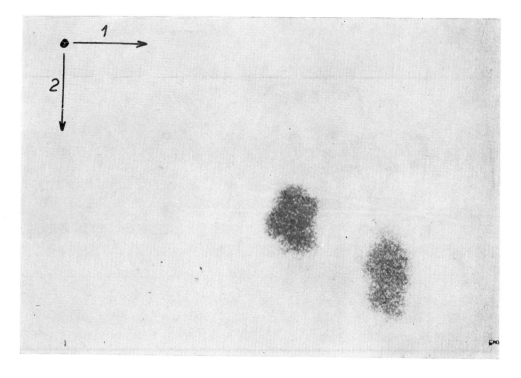

Fig. 19. Bi-dimensional chromatogram of alanine (Ala) and GABA spots after 8 hr hydrolysis in 6 N HCl.

experiments we investigated GABA in the brain following the local application of chlorides of the above ions. Thirty minutes action of 3 or 0.3 M solutions of rubidium, cesium or ammonium chlorides produced a similar rise in GABA in experimental cortices as the application of KCl (results summarized in table 24).

Comparing on the one hand the rise in GABA and on the other hand the rise in lactic acid, it was striking that the rise in GABA was higher the more the lactic acid level of the brain rose. When the rise in lactic acid and GABA was correlated, a positive correlation between them was found ($r = + 0.653 \pm 0.06$).

When lactic acid in the brain rose on an average of 164 μmoles/g N$_2$, GABA rose on an average of 47 μmoles/g N$_2$. The rise in GABA was found not only when endogenous lactic acid in the brain was increased but also after application of exogenous

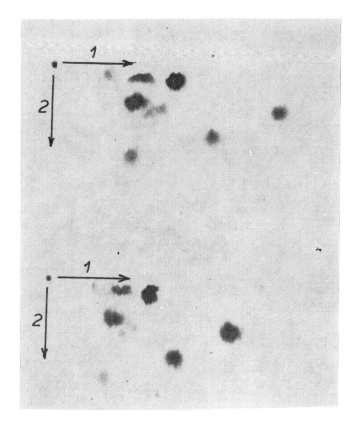

Fig. 20. Bi-dimensional chromatogram of ethanol extract of rat brain cortex following 30 min KCl application (upper part) and the same extract to which 5 μg of α-alanine and 5 μg of GABA were added. 1 — n-But. — ac. ac. — H$_2$O = 4 : 1 : 3; 2 — Pyr. — n-But. — H$_2$O = 5 : 5 : 2.

lactic acid onto the cerebral cortex. A 0.3 M solution of racemic lactic acid applied for 30 min to the ischemic cortex caused an increase in GABA from 97 ± 3 μmoles/g N$_2$ to 134 ± 9 μmoles/g N$_2$ ($n = 8$, $P < 0.01$). However, 0.1 N HCl applied onto the brain cortex did not cause any changes of GABA level in the experimental cortex.

When, on the other hand, we applied GABA to the brain in a 1 M concentration, we found in the cortex of the experimental hemispheres a decrease in glycogen by 56 μmoles/g N$_2$, glucose by 27 μmoles/g N$_2$ and a rise in lactic acid by 134 μmoles/g N$_2$.

The rise in GABA in the cortex with EEG depression is illustrated in figure 18.

Table 24

	I		II		III		IV	
	C	E	C	E	C	E	C	E
3 M	08 ± 5.7	186 ± 10	120 ± 3.2	175 ± 7	111 ± 4	168 ± 7.7	128 ± 4	228 ± 15.2
	$n = 40$		$n = 6$		$n = 6$		$n = 13$	
	$P < 0.01$		$P < 0.01$		$P < 0.01$		$P < 0.01$	
0.3 M	104 ± 7	177 ± 9	112 ± 3	171 ± 9.1	121 ± 2	166 ± 8.8	100 ± 3	154 ± 9
	$n = 10$		$n = 6$		$n = 6$		$n = 6$	
	$P < 0.01$		$P < 0.01$		$P < 0.01$		$P < 0.01$	

The effect of topical application of 3 and 0.3 M solutions of KCl (I), RbCl (II), CsCl (III) and NH$_4$Cl (IV) for 30 min on GABA level in the rat brain cortex. Ligated carotid arteries. Results are expressed in μmoles as M $\pm$ S. E. M./g N$_2$. C — control cortex, E — experimental cortex. n — — number of experiments.

The subsequent figure 19 demonstrates that even 8 hr hydrolysis of the substances described as GABA and alanine with 6 N HCl, which were eluated after previous chromatography, gave only one spot on a two-dimensional chromatogram; it can thus be claimed that GABA itself and not its peptide increased in the brain during the action of K$^+$ions. Also, addition of GABA to extract of the cortex and subsequent bi-dimensional chromatography showed that the mobility of the substance described as GABA was the same as that of added GABA (fig. 20).

C) α-ALANINE IN THE CEREBRAL CORTEX DURING DEPOLARIZATION ASSOCIATED WITH EEG DEPRESSION

Alanine is found in the brain in two forms: as α- and β-alanine. While α-alanine is in brain in concentrations of $8-12$ mg%, β-alanine is found only in traces (Folch-Pi and Le Baron 1957). α-Alanine, on which we focussed our attention, is formed in the brain by transamination of glutamic and aspartic to pyruvic acid, as apparent from the presence of transaminases of both amino acids in the brain (Greenberg 1951, Awapara and Seale 1952, McIlwain 1959). Other forms of α-alanine formation in the brain, such as direct reductive amination of pyruvate found in other tissues (Kaplanskiy and Berezovskaya 1958, Pyatnickaya 1960), were not confirmed so far.

The formation of α-alanine by transamination of dicarboxylic amino acids to pyruvic acid is considered a process which may regulate the rate of the tricarboxylic acid cycle by supplying metabolites for the latter, the utilization of pyruvate and influence the production of lactic acid; as due to the formation of alanine the possibility of anaerobic oxidation of reduced NAD triosephosphate dehydrogenase is in this way limited (Braunstein 1947, 1957).

Experiments *in vitro* have shown that the production of α-alanine is proportional to the amount of pyruvate added to the incubation medium (Kritzmann 1938, Cohen 1939). Our experiments showed that as a result of different stimuli applied to the brain cortex the lactic acid level, a precursor of which is pyruvate, was always increased. It could therefore be expected that in the brain during enhanced glycolysis accompanying EEG depression following ligature of the carotid arteries a part of the pyruvic acid would be transformed to alanine, in particular also because under these experimental conditions the level of dicarboxylic amino acids in the cortex with EEG depression was decreased.

It was found that when no stimuli were applied to the brain, there was no difference in the alanine content between the right and left hemispheres of the same animal. Nor did we find any differences between the cortex of animals with intact carotid arteries and the cortex 30 min after ligature. While in experiments with an intact circulation values of 48 and 49 μmoles/g N_2 resp. were recorded, in experiments after 30 min ligature of the carotid arteries the corresponding values were 50 and 52 μmoles/g N_2 resp. In the brain with an intact circulation EEG depression did not lead to any changes in the alanine level which remained unaltered even after 30 min EEG depression (48 and 50 μmoles /g N_2 resp.).

The application of a 3 M solution of KCl to the ischemic brain for 30 min led to a significant rise in alanine in the experimental hemispheres (from 46 $\pm$ 3.3 μmoles/g N_2 to 89 $\pm$ 4.3 μmoles/g N_2).

In order to rule out the direct influence of exogenous KCl on the rise in alanine (Rybová 1961), we used for our analyses the cortex of the experimental hemisphere divided into two parts: the first to which KCl was applied and the second through which waves of negativity only passed. It was found that in both portions the alanine rose equally. In the portion under the direct influence of KCl it rose from a control level of 43 $\pm$ 2.7 μmoles/g N_2 to 77 $\pm$ 2.8 μmoles/g N_2 and in the portion through which waves of negativity passed to 79 $\pm$ 5 μmoles/g N_2 ($n = 20$, $P < 0.01$).

When after 30 min action of 3 M KCl on the ischemic brain the trachea was compressed for 60 sec, alanine increased in the control as well as in experimental hemispheres. In the control hemisphere to 68 $\pm$ 7 μmoles/g N_2 and in the experimental hemisphere to 128 $\pm$ 12 μmoles/g N_2; ($n = 21$, $P < 0.01$). Also after 150 min asphyxia the differences in the alanine content between the control and experimental hemispheres persisted, whereby the alanine in the control hemisphere rose to 83 $\pm$ 5.5 μmoles/g N_2 and in the experimental one to 149 $\pm$ 16 μmoles/g N_2 ($n = 10$, $P < 0.01$). As compared with values without compression of the trachea, in both instances following asphyxia the rise in the alanine was statistically significant also in the control hemisphere ($P < 0.01$).

The increase in alanine caused by KCl during persisting ligature of the carotid arteries was an irreversible process. When 30 min exposure to 3 M KCl was followed by 30 min restitution, the same differences in alanine content between control and experimental hemispheres as after 30 min exposure to KCl alone were preserved. In the controls 47 ± 3 μmoles/g N_2 alanine and in the experimental hemispheres 91 ± 3.2 μmoles/g N_2 ($n = 10$, $P < 0.01$) were found. Ninety minute restitution with the carotid arteries ligatured caused the disappearance of statistically significant differences between the control and experimental hemispheres because the alanine level increased markedly in both hemispheres. Alanine in the control hemispheres rose to 199 ± 26 μmoles/g N_2 and in the experimental hemispheres to 238 ± 39 μmoles/g N_2 ($n = 7$, $P < 0.3$). Even when the absolute rise in both hemispheres was equal and the difference between the control and experimental hemispheres was maintained, due to the great spread of the results the difference between the two hemispheres was not statistically significant. Thirty minute restitution with the renewed blood supply, which followed after 30 min exposure to 3 M KCl on the ischemic brain, did not abolish the differences between control and experimental hemispheres. In the control hemispheres the alanine level was 53 ± 4 μmoles/g N_2 and in the experimental ones 76 ± 6.6 μmoles/g N_2 ($n = 7$, $P < 0.02$). Only after 90 min restitution with the renewed circulation did the differences between the control and the experimental hemispheres disappear (42 ± 3.1 and 45 ± 3.3 μmoles alanine/g N_2 resp.; $n = 10$, $P < 0.5$).

Since not only 3 M solutions of KCl but also other alkali metals caused a rise in lactic acid in the ischemic cortex, it was expected that the latter would also lead to a rise in alanine. As can be seen from table 25, also after 30 min topical application of 3 and 0.3 M solutions of rubidium, cesium and ammonium chlorides, a significant rise in alanine in the cortex of the experimental hemispheres occurred.

The increase in alanine in the ischemic brain was parallel with that of lactic acid and the higher the lactic acid level the greater also was the increase in alanine. When

Table 25

	I		II		III		IV	
	C	E	C	E	C	E	C	E
3 M	46 ± 3.3	89 ± 4.3	45 ± 3	74 ± 2.2	49 ± 4.9	79 ± 5	44 ± 2.2	76 ± 4
		$n = 40$		$n = 6$		$n = 6$		$n = 13$
		$P < 0.01$		$P < 0.01$		$P < 0.01$		$P < 0.01$
0.3 M	52 ± 5	91 ± 9.5	48 ± 2.8	75 ± 2	54 ± 3	79 ± 2.7	55 ± 3.2	96 ± 9.8
		$n = 10$		$n = 6$		$n = 6$		$n = 6$
		$P < 0.01$		$P < 0.01$		$P < 0.01$		$P < 0.01$

The effect of topical application of 3 and 0.3 M solutions of KCl (I), RbCl (II), CsCl (III) and NH$_4$Cl (IV) for 30 min on α-alanine level in the rat brain cortex. Ligated carotid arteries. Results are expressed in μmoles as M $\pm$ S. E. M./g N_2. C — control cortex, E — experimental cortex. n — number of experiments.

lactic acid increased on an average of 164 ± 13 μmoles/g N₂, the alanine level rose simultaneously by 30.5 ± 2.8 μmoles/g N₂ ($n = 40$, $r = + 0.722$). Alanine rose not only after an increase in endogenous lactic acid in the brain but also after the topical application of a 0.3 M solution of racemic lactic acid to the ischemic brain. Thirty minutes after application of lactic acid alanine in the experimental hemisphere rose from an average of 52 ± 2.7 μmoles/g N₂ to 92 ± 4 μmoles/g N₂ ($n = 8$, $P < 0.01$). Also after the local application of 0.3 M sodium pyruvate alanine rose from 53 ± 2.8 to 92 ± 5.5 μmoles/g N₂ ($n = 6$, $P < 0.01$).

All results submitted in this chapter indicate that under conditions of a reduced blood supply in the brain cortex as a result of depolarization a decrease in dicarboxylic amino acids occurs; this may either be due to their reduced production or to an increased utilization in metabolic processes. In our opinion the reason for their lower level is the increased utilization of amino acids in the oxidative metabolism of the brain. This conclusion was based on our own findings as well as on work with insulin hypoglycemia (Dawson 1950, Cravioto, Massieu and Izquierdo 1951, Massieu et al. 1962), intoxication with fluoroacetate (Awapara 1952, Dawson 1955, Strecker 1957) and on results obtained during convulsive activity of the CNS (Waelsch 1951, Bukin 1959); in all these instances a decrease in glutamic acid in the brain was found due to its higher utilization in energy processes. The decrease in glutamine is in our opinion due to its reduced synthesis; as glutamine synthesis is an exergonic process (Greenberg 1951, Coon and Robinson 1958) and energy produced under conditions of ischemia is according to our concepts used mainly for active ion transport, there is less energy available for the synthesis of glutamine.

The dicarboxylic amino acids are probably utilized due to the slower conversion of isocitric to oxalsuccinic acid, because the activity of isocitric acid dehydrogenase is most sensitive to oxygen deficiency (Kleinzeller 1954).

Amino groups of dicarboxylic amino acids were again found mainly in other amino acids. If we compare our results we can see that a substantial portion of amino groups of glutamic acid, glutamine and aspartic acid appeared in the form of an increased level of alanine and γ-aminobutyrate. This finding confirmed the assumption that the decrease in amino group of one amino acid leads to a rise in another amino acid (McIlwain 1959).

It was found that the mobility of ninhydrin positive substances which increased after application of potassium ions was identical with that of α-alanine and γ-aminobutyric acid in different systems (figs 19, 20).

It was noteworthy that during the rise in lactic acid in the brain and muscles a significant increase in the alanine fraction occurred with a simultaneous decrease in glutamic acid (Ruščák 1961). At the same time it was found that the absolute increase in alanine was the greater the more lactic acid was formed in tissue or the longer glycolysis persisted. Because pyruvic acid is an intermediary product of glycolysis, we can assume that, similarly as in experiments *in vitro* when after the rise of pyruvate in the medium the alanine formation increased (Kritzmann 1938, Cohen 1939), also *in situ* the intensity of pyruvic acid production determines the intensity of its transamination with glutamic acid, the latter being used in energy processes. Experiments with muscles have shown (Ruščák 1962) that for the formation of alanine the period of carbohydrate breakdown is decisive when lactic acid is formed and not the period of restitution when lactic acid disappears. A higher increase in alanine in the brain, as compared with muscles, although the glycolysis was lower, can be explained by the fact that in the brain the glutamic acid concentration is 6−7 times greater and that it acts mainly as a regulator of the cerebral metabolism (Klein 1956, Waelsch 1957).

It is likely that the thus produced alanine is also an important factor participating in the regulation of pH of tissues. This view is supported by our results where we proved a high positive correlation coefficient between the rise in lactate on the one hand and the rise in alanine in tissue on the other hand. Similarly as in our experiments an increase in alanine is also described in nervous tissue of animals where so-called clinical death was produced (Gaevskaya and Nosova 1963), or following a long lasting status epilepticus induced in dogs by administration of penthylentetrazole (Whisler, Tews and Stone 1968). As in all instances in addition to a rise in lactate depolarization of tissue and penetration of Na^+ into cells is also found, it is very probable that the rise in intracellular sodium plays an important role in the rise in alanine in excitable tissue. The increase in alanine could also be caused by a very low level of oxalacetic acid which was not found in our material in detectable amounts. This view is also supported by the findings of Balázs (1965) who demonstrated that in the presence of pyruvate and traces of oxalacetate mitochondria utilize glutamic acid predominantly via transamination with pyruvate.

Glutamate-pyruvate transamination in the CNS plays an important role in the regulation of its metabolism. By the production of alanine the formation of lactic acid is inhibited (Weil-Malherbe 1938) and thus the tissue pH variations diminished; moreover, amino groups are preserved for rebuilding the altered amino acid component of tissue (Braunstein 1947) and at the same time α-oxoglutaric acid is formed, which has a catalytic effect on pyruvate oxidation (Kleinzeller 1954) as well as alanine which can be readily utilized by nervous tissue in energy yielding processes (Mullins 1953).

Price (1961) who described an increase in alanine in muscles of houseflies after their stimulation considered the formation of α-alanine in tissue as a reaction which is equivalent to the formation of lactate: in this reaction reduced NAD is also oxidized. By transamination glutamate-pyruvate α-oxoglutarate is obtained which can be transformed by reductive amination to glutamate and this way NADH is oxidized:

$$Pyr + Glu \rightarrow Ala + \alpha\text{-}OG,$$
$$\alpha\text{-}OG + NADH + NH_3 \rightarrow Glu + NAD + H_2O.$$

The resulting reaction then is: $Pyr + NADH + NH_3 \rightarrow Ala + NAD$.

102

It is probable that transamination glutamate-pyruvate with a marked decrease in glutamic acid and rise in alanine is found only when the supply of energy sources to the brain is reduced and tissues utilize mainly their own energy reserves. This explains the alanine formation in our experiments as well as the results of Gaevskaya and Nosova (1963) who recorded a marked rise in alanine in the brain following asphyxia or decapitation of animals. A greater turnover of alanine under conditions when its stationary level in the brain remains unchanged in spite of a higher rate of ion movements is not excluded but could be proved only in experiments with labelled compounds.

The increase in GABA can be explained by several factors. Since we assume that due to agents evoking EEG depression the observed negativity waves are associated with a rise in extracellular potassium similarly as in experiments with an intact circulation (Křivánek and Bureš 1960, Brinley, Kandel and Marshall 1960) the rise in GABA can be explained, as demonstrated in experiments *in vitro* (Kini and Quastel 1959, Rybová 1960), by the influence of an increased level of extracellular potassium which enhances the transformation of glutamic acid to GABA. This assumption is supported to a certain extent by experiments with the application of rubidium, cesium and ammonium chlorides which exert a similar metabolic effect as potassium and also evoke EEG depression (Bessman and Lardy 1952, Weil-Malherbe 1956, Marshall 1959, Hertz and Schou 1962), the application of which leads to a rise in GABA even when 0.3 M solutions were used and when sodium and lithium chlorides in the same concentration did not influence the GABA level in brain (Ruščák 1962).

Further reason for the rise in GABA could be an increase in lactic acid in tissue, which reduces its pH and in this way, similarly as in experiments *in vitro* (Roberts and Baxter 1960), glutamic acid decarboxylase activity could be increased: thus the rise in GABA would be the result of its higher production due to a lowered tissue pH. We cannot rule out as a further reason of GABA increase also α-oxoglutarate deficiency. We noted its declining trend in our experiments and it is known that the utilization of GABA proceeds via transamination with α-oxoglutaric acid (Cacioppo, Pandolfo and di Chiara 1959, Wilson, Hill and Koeppe 1959, Roberts and Baxter 1960).

Although from our experiments we cannot define precisely the reason for GABA increase, its position in the brain metabolism seems to be more elucidated. We assume that our experiments have proved the homeostatic function of GABA in the brain which was already supposed by some authors previously (Roberts and Baxter 1960, Udenfriend, Weissbach and Mitoma 1960), as we demonstrated that there exists a direct relationship between the rise in lactic acid and GABA. We assume that the rise in GABA in the brain, similarly as the rise in alanine, is a reaction to the reduced pH in nervous tissue and should contribute to the maintenance of a constant pH in nerve elements (Domonkos and Huszák 1959). The enhanced glycolysis by exogenous GABA can, on the other hand, be conceived as a response to the higher pH due to γ-aminobutyric acid, as it is known that a rise in pH above physiological levels enhances glycolysis (Birmingham and Elliot 1949).

The EEG record (fig. 21) indicated that while during the EEG depression the electrical activity of the cortex also declined, 30 min after removal of KCl it approached, even when the carotids were ligatured, the initial value, despite the fact that the GABA level was at that time significantly higher than before the application of KCl. The specific inhibitory function of GABA in the CNS appears therefore improbable; on the other hand, Roberts and Kuriyama (1968) in a review article suggest that GABA can be an inhibitory transmitter in at least some synapses.

The unaltered stationary amino acid level during intact cerebral circulation can be explained by the fact that although the amino acid component we investigated is utilized in metabolic processes, it is rapidly renewed via the amination of α-keto acids of tricarboxylic acid cycle and therefore labelled compounds would have to be used to resolve this problem.

As far as the connection between cell elements and the level of the investigated amino acids in the brain is concerned, we found that except for a decrease in γ-aminobutyric acid (table 26) there are no differences in the amino acid content between intact cortex and cortex with a relative predominance of non-nerve elements. This finding suggests that the utilization of glutamic acid via the GABA shunt depends only on nerve cells and is in agreement with the data of van Gelder (1965) who detected enzymes of the so-called "GABA shunt" only in nerve cells. That the metabolism of glutamate via the GABA shunt is bound only to nerve elements is suggested also by further results of ours, where we found a lower glutamate decarboxylase activity in tissue with a relative predominance of non-nerve elements, obtained by the procedure described in chapter 2. While we recorded in homogenates of intact cortex after 1 hr incubation in an atmosphere of N_2 with 50 mM glutamic acid + 0.5 mM pyridoxal phosphate a GABA increase of 95 ± 6 μmoles/g N_2 in cortex with an approximate 20 % reduction of nerve cells the GABA increase was only

Table 26

	C	E
Glu	402 ± 18	404 ± 14
Asp	294 ± 9	280 ± 11
GABA	123 ± 9.9	98 ± 11.3
Ala	47 ± 1.7	50 ± 2.2

Glutamate (Glu), aspartate (Asp), γ-aminobutyrate (GABA) and α-alanine (Ala) in the control cortex (C) and the cortex with relative predominance of non-nerve cells (E) in rats in μmoles as $M \pm S. E. M/g N_2$. Mean values of 12 experiments.

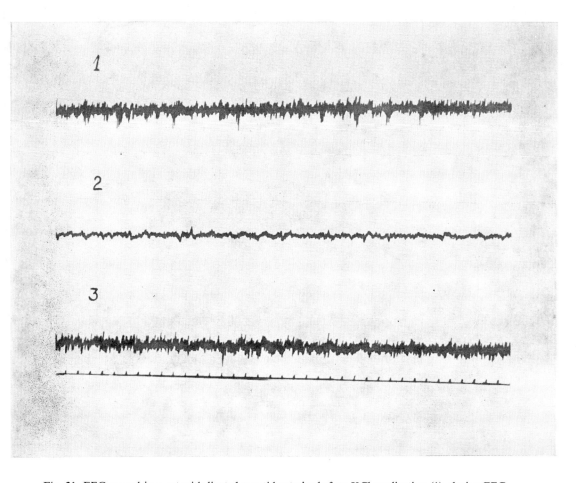

Fig. 21. EEG record in a rat with ligated carotid arteries before KCl application (1), during EEG depression (2) and 30 min after washing off KCl (3).

75 ± 4.8 μmoles/g N_2 ($n = 10$, $P < 0.05$). Also the uptake of GABA by slices *in vitro* was lower in preparations with a relative reduction of nerve cells. While in the controls after 1 hr incubation in Krebs-Ringer phosphate solution in an atmosphere of O_2 with a substrate of 10 mM glucose and 1 mM GABA the resulting GABA concentration was 396 ± 22 μmoles/g N_2, in slices with a relative predominance of glia the GABA level was only 300 ± 16 μmoles/g N_2 ($n = 6$, $P < 0.02$). The presented results provide in our opinion evidence that while the metabolism of other amino acids is uniformly distributed between nerve and non-nerve elements, the metabolism of glutamate via the GABA shunt depends on nerve cells only.

105

FORMATION OF α-ALANINE IN THE RAT BRAIN AT CELLULAR AND SUBCELLULAR LEVELS IN RELATION TO pH AND IONIC COMPOSITION OF THE MEDIUM

Prolonged depolarization of rat brain cortex associated with EEG depression during ligature of the carotid arteries led to a rise in ninhydrin-positive [substance (Ruščák 1963), further analyses of which showed that it was α-alanine. Later also van Harreveld and Kooiman (1965) described during the EEG depression wave the release of ninhydrin-positive substances into the fluid washing the brain surface; the di-nitro-fluorbenzene derivatives of one of them displayed on chromatographic analyses the same mobility as α-alanine. Gaevskaya and Nosova (1962) observed the increase of α-alanine in dog brain by so-called clinical death and Whisler, Tews and Stone (1968) following long lasting seizure activity. It may therefore be assumed that any depolarization of nervous tissue *in situ* is followed, similarly as *in vitro* (Kini and Quastel 1959, Rybová 1961), by a shift of metabolic processes towards reactions which lead among others to an increased α-alanine formation in tissue. α-Alanine which is a product of transamination of glutamate with pyruvate (Chain et al. 1962, Ruščák and Macejová 1965, Balázs 1965) inhibits, moreover, in a concentration of $20-100$ $\mu g/ml$ significantly the stimulation of the superior cervical ganglion of the cat by potassium or acetylcholine (Damjanovich et al. 1960). An increased formation of α-alanine in relation to the polarity of nervous tissue, the dependence of its production on the simultaneous utilization of carbohydrates and glutamic acid in oxidative processes and its inhibitory effect on the activity of nerve structures made us investigate in greater detail the production of α-alanine at cellular and subcellular levels and in further experiments also the influence of L-α-alanine on the metabolism of nervous tissue *in vitro*.

The first experiments were performed on cortex slices or homogenates of rats, incubated in Krebs-Ringer phosphate solution in Warburg manometric flasks in an atmosphere of air or O_2 for 1 hr at 37 °C after 15 min preincubation in 0.15 M Tris-HCl, pH 7.4, at O °C, with the following substrates: glutamic acid, glutamic acid + α-oxoglutaric acid, pyruvic acid + glutamic acid, pyruvic acid and glucose. All substrates had a concentration of 3 mM except glucose, the concentration of which was 6.6 mM; the pH of the media was 6.2, 7.4 and 8.6. After the incubation the slices were subjected to repeated extractions with 70 % ethanol and the extracted free amino acids were estimated by one-dimensional paper chromatography in a system n-butanol—acetic acid—water (12 : 3 : 5) or by electrophoresis (Mikeš 1957) in combination with chromatography.

It was found that the utilization of endogenous sources even without the addition of substrate was relatively high, as evident from the average O_2 consumption -1550 $\mu moles$ per g N_2/hr. The addition of any of the above-mentioned substrates led to a higher O_2 consumption, the highest O_2 consumption being in experiments with pyruvate.

In slices to which no substrate was added the alanine level was 14.3 $\mu moles/g$ N_2. When we added glutamic acid only or in combination with α-oxoglutaric acid we obtained alanine values of $31-44$ $\mu moles$ per g N_2. The increase in alanine, as compared with experiments without addition of substrate, was in all experiments highly significant. When pyruvic acid was used as substrate, the rise in alanine in the slices

109

was much greater than after glutamic acid or glutamic acid + α-oxoglutaric acid resp. The results also showed that with pyruvic acid as substrate α-alanine in the slices rose with the increasing pH of the medium, i.e. at an acid pH the alanine level in slices was lower than in an alkaline one. The rise in alanine in the group with pyruvic acid and pyruvic + glutamic acid, as compared with the groups without pyruvic acid, was also statistically significant. Glucose alone maintained in the slices the same alanine level as glutamic acid or glutamic acid combined with α-oxoglutarate. The addition of glutamic acid to glucose medium, however, led to a significant rise in alanine in the slices. (For summarized results see table 27.)

In subsequent experiments we paid attention not only to the relationship between alanine formation and the substrates used but also in relation to the intensity of the metabolism. Because it has been proved that an intense metabolism in nervous tissue depends on the mutual equilibrium of mono- and bivalent cations (Gonda and Quastel 1962, Whittam 1962, Hertz and Schou 1962, Whittam 1964, Ruščák and Whittam 1967), we decided also to investigate the formation of alanine in nervous tissue under conditions of different metabolic intensity. The cortical slices of rats were in-

Table 27

Substrate	pH of the medium	O_2	Ala	n
none	7.4	1550 ± 80	14.3 ± 1.9	8
Glu	6.2	2002 ± 99	44.0 ± 4.8	10
	7.4	2130 ± 121	31.5 ± 2.6	8
	8.6	2110 ± 115	37.0 ± 3.9	8
Glu + α − OG	6.2	2137 ± 118	44.5 ± 1.9	9
	7.4	2291 ± 103	31.2 ± 1.4	7
	8.6	1995 ± 176	35.6 ± 4.0	8
Pyr	6.2	2350 ± 144	69.0 ± 5.5	10
	7.4	2418 ± 132	51.7 ± 2.3	8
	8.6	2634 ± 165	96.4 ± 7.9	8
Pyr + Glu	7.4	2850 ± 147	101.0 ± 7.2	8
	8.6	2626 ± 133	125.4 ± 11.4	8
Glc	7.4	2041 ± 133	28.1 ± 1.2	8
Glc + Glu	7.4	2501 ± 127	78.5 ± 4.5	17

Oxygen consumption (O_2) and α-alanine formation (Ala) in μmoles as M ± S. E. M./g N_2 in the rat brain cortex slices incubated in Krebs-Ringer phosphate solution in the air atmosphere at different pH with various substrates. Glu—L-glutamic acid 3 mM, OG—α-oxoglutaric acid 3 mM, Pyr—pyruvic acid 3 mM, Glc — glucose 6.6 mM. n — number of experiments.

110

cubated in Warburg flasks in an atmosphere of O_2 at 37 °C for 1 hr in a Krebs-Ringer phosphate solution with 4 mM L-glutamate and 4 mM pyruvate as substrates and other slices in a solution where sodium was replaced by an equivalent amount of potassium salts. In a pure potassium medium after 1 hr incubation a lower O_2 consumption was recorded (a decrease from 88 ± 1.9 to 67 ± 3.2 μmoles/g wet wt, $n = 10$), as well as a lower alanine level. In slices incubated in a so-called balanced medium 51 ± 2.3 μmoles alanine/g N_2 were found, while in the slices from a pure potassium medium only 34 ± 2 μmoles alanine/g N_2 ($n = 10$). Because the observed differences may have been conditioned by lower levels of substrates in the slices in a pure potassium medium (e. g. glutamic acid in slices from the balanced medium was found in a concentration of 1.1 mM/g N_2 and in the potassium medium only 0.37 mM/g N_2), as well as by possible escape of alanine from the slices into the medium, we investigated the effect of monovalent cations on α-alanine formation also in homogenates under aerobic and under anaerobic conditions.

When homogenates from rat brain cortex slices preincubated in Tris at 0 °C were incubated in a medium containing 3 mM $CaCl_2$, 3 mM $MgCl_2$, 4 mM L-glutamate + 4 mM pyruvate, 0.25 mM pyridoxal-5-phosphate, 6 mM ATP, 2 mM NAD, 20 mM phosphate buffer and 75 mM NaCl + 59 mM KCl or when instead of NaCl only KCl was used, a higher O_2 consumption as well as higher alanine formation in the medium containing sodium + potassium were observed. The O_2 consumption in the pure potassium medium decreased, as compared with the sodium medium, from 80 ± 2.2 to 66 ± 2.1 μmoles O_2/g tissue wet wt and the alanine formation declined from 383 ± 29 to 219 ± 9 μmoles/g N_2 after 1 hr incubation ($n = 10$, $P < 0.01$).

From the hitherto presented results it may be concluded that the formation of alanine is conditioned by the rate of utilization of glutamic acid in oxidative processes and that these processes are probably in a close relationship, as they depend on the presence of $Na^+ + K^+$, with metabolic processes regulated by membrane ATP-ase.

When homogenates were, incubated for 1 hr in an atmosphere of N_2, sodium also enhanced the alanine formation. While in homogenates incubated in a pure potassium medium 2913 ± 57 μmoles alanine/g N_2 were present, in a medium containing also sodium 3689 ± 39 μmoles alanine/g N_2 were found.

Because a substantial part of energy produced by the nervous tissue is used to maintain the electrochemical gradient which can be influenced by ouabain, we decided to investigate in subsequent experiments the influence of ouabain on alanine production as well as on that of other amino acids. After 1 hr incubation of brain cortex homogenates the O_2 consumption in the controls was 80 ± 1.9 and in homogenates with addition of ouabain with a final concentration of 20 μM 62 ± 1.1 μmoles O_2/g tissue wet wt. Although the O_2 consumption of homogenates without ouabain was higher, we did not find any differences in the alanine content between the two groups (360 μmoles/g N_2 in the medium without ouabain and 357 μmoles/g

N$_2$ in the medium with ouabain). In the medium without ouabain the resulting production of aspartic acid was, however, higher (164 ± 6.8 μmoles/g N$_2$ as compared with 142 ± 5.1 μmoles/g N$_2$; $n = 6$, $P < 0.05$), but GABA formation was higher in the presence of ouabain (113 ± 8.4 as compared with 137 ± 6.2 μmoles/g N$_2$; $n = 6$, $P < 0.05$). We did not confirm the data of Gonda and Quastel (1962) that ouabain suppressed alanine formation and did not influence the formation of aspartic acid and GABA; if one considers the unaltered amount of alanine but a lower O$_2$ consumption it seems rather that ouabain stimulated alanine formation despite the lowered metabolic level.

The results of the above experiments showed that the formation of alanine in slices depended on the pH as well as on the ionic composition of the medium and the utilized substrates. When glutamic acid was used as the substrate in combination with pyruvate or glucose, the glycolysis of which is stimulated in the presence of glutamic acid (McIlwain 1959), a higher alanine production was found; this finding may be considered as evidence of the enhanced utilization of glutamate by transamination with pyruvate. Similar results were obtained by Beloff-Chain et al. (1962) who found by means of 3 − ^{14}C-labelled pyruvate added to cortical slices a high amination of pyruvate to alanine. The higher production of alanine in an alkaline medium was probably due to the higher activity of glutamate-pyruvate transaminase in this medium as can be assumed from the results of Hopper and Segal (1964) who found that the optimum pH of this enzyme in liver was in alkaline medium. It is, however, also possible that a higher alanine production in an alkaline medium is the result of a raised metabolic level at which glutamic acid utilization could be enhanced. This possibility is suggested not only by a rise in alanine but also in GABA (Kometiani 1965, Ruščák and Macejová 1965) in an alkaline medium due to the enhanced glutamic acid utilization via the GABA shunt. The primary role of the metabolic intensity on alanine production is also suggested by our experiments where we found under aerobic conditions more alanine in a medium containing Na$^+$ and K$^+$; the formation of alanine under aerobic conditions was stimulated by sodium, while in anaerobic conditions sodium inhibited the formation of alanine. It thus seems very probable that there can exist in addition to the metabolic intensity also some subcellular structures where sodium chloride exerts a different effect on α-alanine formation.

The high O$_2$ consumption with glutamate + pyruvate as the substrates provides further evidence that the transamination glutamate-pyruvate is in addition to the transamination glutamate-oxalacetate (Krebs and Bellamy 1960) the second main pathway of oxidation of glutamic acid also in nervous tissue similarly as in other tissues (Klingenberg 1963). Pyruvate stimulates the transfer of the amino group from glutamic to pyruvic acid and thus promotes the oxidation of glutamic acid similarly as glucose (Sellinger et al. 1962, Balázs 1965).

The alanine formation in subcellular structures was followed after 1 hr incubation of fractions prepared as described earlier. These were incubated in an atmosphere of N_2, in media containing glutamic acid 20 mM, pyruvic acid 10 mM, pyridoxal-5-phosphate 2 mM and phosphate buffer pH 7.4 20 mM or Tris-HCl buffer pH 7.4 60 mM. Alanine was estimated, similarly as in experiments with slices and homogenates, by separation on paper as well as on a Dowex 2 × 8 column in the acetate cycle and by colorimetric determination of the produced alanine according to the method of Moore and Stein (1954), or enzymatically according to Swick, Barnstein and Stange (1965). The results are presented in μmoles of alanine/g prot. contained in the sediment after denaturation of proteins as the arithmetical mean $\pm$ S. E. M.

Alanine was formed in all subcellular structures except microsomes, as can be seen from the results given in table 28.

Table 28

CM	My	Ne$_1$	Ne$_2$	Mi	Me	Ms	S
860 $\pm$ 18	306 $\pm$ 11	442 $\pm$ 44	478 $\pm$ 32	2484 $\pm$ 40	560 $\pm$ 26	0	3422 $\pm$ 86

α-Alanine formation in μmoles as M $\pm$ S. E. M./g prot. in the crude mitochondrial fraction (CM), myelin fraction (My), nerve ending fractions (Ne$_1$ and Ne$_2$), mitochondrial fraction (Mi), membrane fraction (Me), microsomal fraction (Ms) and the soluble fraction (S) after 1 hr incubation.

Table 29

C	I	II	III	IV
+ NaCl 140 mM	2667 $\pm$ 89	2546 $\pm$ 118	2520 $\pm$ 56	2200 $\pm$ 32
+ KCl 140 mM	1820 $\pm$ 92	1804 $\pm$ 96	2444 $\pm$ 49	2290 $\pm$ 49
	1550 $\pm$ 62	1270 $\pm$ 112	2534 $\pm$ 66	2185 $\pm$ 47

α-Alanine formation in μmoles as M $\pm$ S. E. M./g prot. in mitochondria of gray matter (I), mitochondria of white matter (II), soluble fraction of gray matter (III) and soluble fraction of white matter (IV) of beef brain after 1 hr incubation in control experiments (C), in the presence of 140 mM NaCl and 140 mM KCl resp. Mean values of 8 experiments. Controls incubated in 20 mM phosphate buffer, pH 7.4.

Since in liver tissue glutamate-alanine transaminase activity was found only in the mitochondrial and in the soluble fraction (Swick, Barnstein and Stange 1965), it was assumed that the alanine formation in other subcellular structures was due to the contamination of the examined sub-fractions either with mitochondria or with particles of cytoplasmic origin.

In beef brain, as regards alanine formation, no differences were found between mitochondrial and soluble fractions from white and gray matter.

The enzymic activity in both fractions was, however, dependent on the effect of Cl^- ions, as well as on the pH of the incubation medium and on the buffer used.

Chloride ions inhibited the alanine formation only in mitochondria but not in the soluble fraction. Potassium chloride exhibited at the same ionic strength a significantly higher inhibitory effect than sodium chloride (see table 29). The inhibitory

effect of Cl⁻ ions started already at a concentration of 80 mM, the half-maximal effect
was observed at 100 mM and the maximal inhibition was attained at 150 mM
(fig. 22).

As regards the pH-optimum of the incubation medium, differences between the
specific activity of both tested fractions were also observed. While in the soluble
fraction a pH-optimum at 7.5 — 8 was reached, as well in Tris as in phosphate buffer,
in the mitochondrial fraction the pH-optimum ranged between 7.5 — 9 (fig. 23).

Maleic acid, suggested to be an alkylating agent of SH-groups of proteins, inhibited the alanine formation in mitochondria at about 60 %, while in the soluble
fraction only at 16 % (fig. 24).

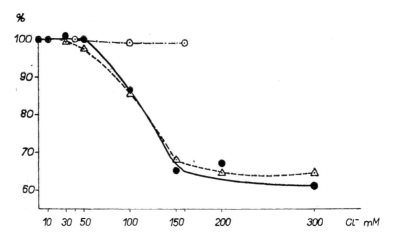

Fig. 22. The relative inhibition of α-alanine formation in relation to Cl⁻ ions. ⊙—⊙, — soluble
fraction; △—△ — membrane fraction; ●—● — mitochondrial fraction. The control values taken
as 100 %.

p-Chloromercuribenzoate, which has a blocking effect on SH-groups, inhibited
the alanine formation to the same extent in both sub-fractions (fig.25).

The enzyme producing α-alanine in mitochondria is firmly bound to mitochondrial
structures and cannot be separated by hyposmotic shock in distilled water. Sonification of the mitochondrial fraction (15 KHz for 2 min) led, however, to the libera-
tion of the enzyme of the mitochondrial structures. After centrifugation of
the sonificated material (220,000 g/hr), two fractions were obtained. The determination of the enzymic activity in both fractions showed that a higher one was present
in the supernatant — 62 μmoles/g prot./min, while in the sediment an activity of
8 μmoles/g prot./min was found. The inhibitory effect of the Cl⁻ ions on the enzymic
activity of the sonificated material remained preserved, as well in the mitochondrial
sediment, as in the supernatant (fig. 26).

As far as the production of alanine is concerned, our findings were similar to
those described by Salganicoff and de Robertis (1965). Neither the above authors

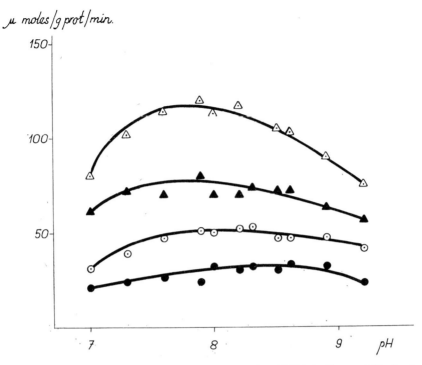

Fig. 23. The effect of pH on α-alanine formation. △—△— 60 mM Tris buffer – soluble fraction; ▲—▲ — 20 mM phosphate buffer – soluble fraction; ⊙—⊙ — 60 mM Tris buffer – mitochondria; ●—● — 20 mM phosphate buffer – mitochondria.

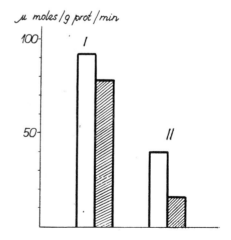

Fig. 24. The inhibition of α-alanine formation in the presence of 100 mM maleic acid. I — soluble fraction; II — mitochondrial fraction. White columnes — control values; striped columnes — experimental values.

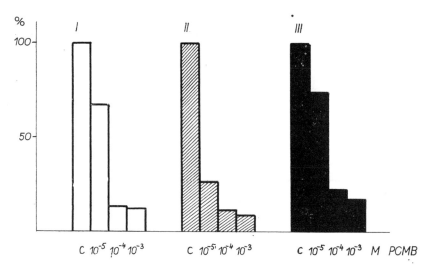

Fig. 25. The relative inhibition of α-alanine formation in the presence of different concentrations of *p*-chlormercuribenzoate sodium. I — mitochondria; II — membrane fraction; III — soluble fraction. Control values (C) taken as 100 %.

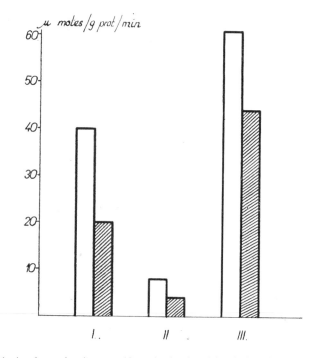

Fig. 26. The α-alanine formation in unsonificated mitochondria (I); in mitochondrial sediment (II) and in the soluble fraction following sonification of mitochondria (III) 2 min 15 kilocycles. White columns — control results; striped columns — in the presence of 140 mM NaCl.

nor we succeeded in localizing the alanine formation in the mitochondria or in the soluble fraction only, as it was done in the liver (Segal, Beattie and Hopper 1962, Hopper and Segall 1964, Swick, Barnstein and Stange 1965).

Since no differences were found between the activity of gray and white matter, it seems probable that all cell types of the CNS are involved in α-alanine production, regardless their origin or morphological differences.

As already mentioned the formation of α-alanine was inhibited by Cl^- ions only in the mitochondrial fraction. Šorm and Turský (1955) described an inhibition of glutamate decarboxylase by Cl^- ions in brain homogenates, but we did not find any similar data as regards glutamate α-alanine transaminase. In our experiments Cl^- ions did not inhibit the activity of mitochondrial glutamate-oxalacetate transaminase, although the enzymic activity of the latter was of a higher order (unpublished data). The inhibitory effect of chloride ions only on mitochondrial glutamate-alanine transaminase can be taken as a proof that the enzyme from the mitochondrial fraction differs in its properties from those occurring in the soluble fraction. Similarly, Cl^- ions inhibited the glutamate-alanine transaminase in liver, heart and kidney cortex mitochondria, but were ineffective in the soluble enzymes (unpublished results).

According to our findings the maximum of alanine production in the soluble fraction at pH 7.5—8 was reached, while in mitochondria such a dependence on the pH of the incubation medium could not be observed. These results do not agree with those of Hopper and Segal (1964), Katunuma et al. (1965), and Swick, Barnstein and Stange 1965, working with liver subcellular particles. The mentioned authors found a typical pH-optimum for the mitochondrial and for the soluble fractions, although different for both sub-fractions. Our results with liver, heart and kidney cortex mitochondria showed the same properties as the brain mitochondria — pH-optimum between 7.5—9, independent on the buffer used (unpublished results).

The different effect of Cl^- ions, the dependence on pH of the incubation medium and the relatively higher effect of maleic acid on mitochondrial alanine formation seem to indicate that in the nerve tissue there are at least two different systems taking part in the α-alanine formation: one being bound to the mitochondria and the other solubilized in the cytoplasm of the cells.

THE EFFECT OF L-α-ALANINE ON O₂ CONSUMPTION AND GLYCOLYSIS BY BRAIN SLICES IN VITRO

During depolarization of the brain cortex induced by EEG depression the alanine concentration in the depolarized tissue was increased. The formation of alanine during EEG depression was directly correlated with the intensity of lactic acid formation in the depolarized cortex. The above facts made us investigate the effect of L-α-alanine on the metabolism of the cortex *in vitro;* we wanted to elucidate whether alanine can influence the metabolism of nervous tissue similarly as ouabain by influencing the activity of membrane ATP-ase (prolongation of depolarization), or whether its possible interference with the metabolism takes place at another site. This question arose not only from our own experiments but also from those of Damjanovich and his co-workers (1960) who found that L-α-alanine in concentrations of 20—100 μg/ml inhibited or completely blocked the excitation in the superior cervical ganglion of the cat evoked by acetylcholine or potassium ions.

The O_2 consumption was estimated in cortex slices of rats, incubated in Krebs-Ringer phosphate solution at pH 7.4 in Warburg manometric flasks at 37 °C in an atmosphere of O_2 for 1 hr with different substrates in the presence of L-α-alanine, as indicated in the following tables. After incubation the material was deproteinized with $HClO_4$ and lactic acid was determined as described above. The activity of membrane-ATP-ase was assayed in the membrane fraction which was incubated in a medium as described by Deul and McIlwain (1961) for 5 min at 37 °C and after deproteinization with $HClO_4$ the split of inorganic phosphorus was determined according to Martin and Doty (1949). The proteins were determined colorimetrically by means of Folin's reagent, beef albumin being used as standard (Mann Res. Lab.).

L-α-alanine in 3—90 mM concentrations with 6.6 mM glucose as substrate did not influence the O_2 consumption and aerobic glycolysis by slices in the medium which contained 5 mM potassium. The O_2 consumption by control slices was 88 ± 3.8 and by slices with 3—90 mM alanine in the medium 90 ± 6 μmoles O_2/g wet wt/hr. After 1 hr incubation we found in the control slices 11.1 ± 1.4 μmoles lactate/g wet wt and in the slices with alanine 12.5 ± 1.4 μmoles/g wet wt. L-glutamic acid even in concentrations of 3 mM caused a rise in O_2 consumption to 108 ± 2 μmoles/g wet wt/hr (n = 11, P < 0.01) and lactic acid rose in the presence of glutamic acid to 23 ± 2.5 μmoles/g wet wt (n = 6, P < 0.01).

When the external K^+ concentration was increased to 105 mM, the glucose concentration being 6.6 mM and that of alanine 30 mM, we observed a significant decrease in O_2 consumption and lactate formation by slices incubated in the presence of alanine. Glutamic acid, on the other hand, did not produce any additive stimulating effect on O_2 consumption when the potassium concentration in the medium was high. When compared with 20 μM ouabain, the inhibition with alanine was by about one-half smaller. 15 and 90 mM alanine had a similar effect as 30 mM alanine (table 30), as regards O_2 consumption and lactate formation.

In order to locate the effect of alanine we proceeded with our experiments along two lines. We assumed that, based on results with other tissues (Quastel 1965), alanine could influence glucose transport from the medium to the tissue and thus due to lack of substrate reduce the O_2 consumption in the stimulated tissue, or it

121

Table 30

	C	P_1	P_2	P_3	P_4
O_2	154 ± 5.3	132 ± 2.7	129 ± 3.7	107 ± 3.5	146 ± 3
	$n = 17$	$n = 17$	$n = 14$	$n = 6$	$n = 10$
		$P < 0.01$	$P < 0.01$	$P < 0.01$	n. s.
LA	38 ± 1.8	32 ± 1.2	—	40 ± 0.09	—
	$n = 5$	$n = 5$	—	$n = 6$	—
		$P < 0.05$	—	n. s.	—

Oxygen consumption (O_2) and lactic acid formation (LA) by rat brain cortex slices incubated 1 hr in Krebs-Ringer phosphate medium pH 7.4, O_2 atmosphere, with elevated potassium level (105 mM KCl) in μmoles as M $\pm$ S. E. M. C— control experiments with 6.6 mM glucose as the substrate, $P_1 +$ 30 mM L-α-alanine, $P_2 +$ 90 mM L-α-alanine, $P_3 +$ 30 μM ouabain, $P_4 +$ 30 mM L-glutamic acid. n — number of experiments, n. s. — differences statistically not significant.

Table 32

C_1	C_2	A	B
0.73 ± 0.03	3.08 ± 0.05	2.98 ± 0.05	2.14 ± 0.05
		$C_2 - A > 0.5$	$C_2 - B < 0.01$

Inorganic phosphate in μmoles as M $\pm$ S. E.M./mg prot./5 min split off after incubation of membranes isolated from rat brain hemispheres in the mediums of following composition : C_1 : Tris-HCl pH 7.4 150 mM + $MgCl_2$ 3 mM + Tris-ATP 6 mM. C_2 : NaCl 100 mM + KCl 20 mM + Tris-HCl pH 7.4 30 mM + $MgCl_2$ 3 mM + Tris-ATP 6 mM. A : $C_2 +$ 30 mM L-α-alanine. B : $C_2 +$ 50 μM ouabain. Mean values of 10 experiments.

could inhibit the activity of transport ATP-ase and thus the entire metabolism. Therefore in subsequent experiments we kept the glucose level in controls unchanged (6.6 mM) but to the slices with alanine glucose was added in a concentration of 17 and 30 mM resp. It was found that with 17 mM glucose the O_2 consumption was still inhibited by alanine; when the glucose was raised to 30 mM no differences in the O_2 consumption of control and experimental slices were observed, not even when the glucose in the controls was increased above 30 mM. In subsequent experiments instead of glucose pyruvate in the presence of 30 mM L-α-alanine was used as substrate. It was found that with this substrate alanine did not inhibit the stimulated O_2 consumption (table 31). Alanine did not influence the O_2 consumption and glycolysis in cortical homogenates in the presence of 105 mM potassium in the medium nor in slices incubated in a sodium-free medium where sodium was replaced by an equimolar amount of choline chloride; with choline chloride in both control and experimental slices, the O_2 consumption was 31 μmoles/g wet wt/hr.

As can be seen from the results listed in table 32, 30 mM L-α-alanine did not exert any effect on the activity of membrane ATP-ase, while 50 μM ouabain reduced it by 30.6 %.

Table 31

	C	G_1	G_2	H	H_1	Pyr	Pyr_1
O_2	154 ± 5.3 $n = 17$	133 ± 6.2 $n = 10$ $P < 0.05$	160 ± 4 $n = 8$ n. s.	78 ± 1.8	80 ± 2.8 $n = 10$ n. s.	161 ± 8	159 ± 7.8 $n = 10$ n. s.
LA	38 ± 1.8 $n = 5$	32.7 ± 1.4 $n = 5$ n. s.	41 ± 3.5 n. s.	14.5 ± 0.3	14.5 ± 0.3 $n = 10$ n. s.	—	—

Oxygen consumption (O_2) and lactic acid formation (LA) by rat brain cortex slices and homogenates in μmoles as $M \pm S. E. M.$/g wet wt/ hr incubated in Krebs-Ringer phosphate medium pH 7.4, O_2 atmosphere, with elevated potassium level in the medium (105 mM KCl). C — control experiments with 6.6 mM glucose, G_1 — glucose 17 mM + 30 mM L-α-alanine, G_2 — glucose 30 mM + L-α-alanine 30 mM, H — homogenates with 6.6 mM glucose, H_1 — homogenates with 6.6 mM glucose + 30 mM L-α-alanine, Pyr — 6.6 mM sodium pyruvate, Pyr_1 — 6.6 mM sodium pyruvate + 30 mM L-α-alanine. n — number of experiments. n. s. — differences statistically not significant.

The above results showed that L-α-alanine had a significant inhibitory effect on the metabolism of cerebral cortex slices with glucose as substrate; this inhibition of O_2 consumption was observed only in tissue, the metabolism of which was stimulated by potassium and the cell membranes were intact. A similar inhibition of the metabolism in stimulated tissue was only observed in the presence of hypnotics and narcotics (Quastel 1959, McIlwain 1959); also ouabain reduced the O_2 consumption only in tissue stimulated by potassium (Gonda and Quastel 1962, Ruščák and Whittam 1967). The decrease in O_2 consumption in brain slices with oligomycin was also greater when there was a high potassium concentration in the incubation medium (Ruščák and Whittam 1967). Contrary to narcotics, hypnotics and oligomycin which act on the metabolism by a block of the electron transport system and ouabain which influences the metabolism by inhibiting the activity of membrane ATP-ase (Quastel 1959, Gonda and Quastel 1962, Minikami, Kakinuma and Yoshikawa 1963, Ruščák and Whittam 1967), alanine reduces the metabolism of brain slices *in vitro* probably by inhibiting the glucose transport to the cells. Evidence of the fact that alanine may reduce the transport of glucose into cells is provided by the data of Quastel (1965) and Hindmarsh, Kilby and Wiseman (1966). Everted intestinal mucosa was able to transport across its epithelium significantly less glucose when amino acids including alanine were added to the incubation medium. We were unable to prove directly the inhi-

123

bition of glucose transport into cortex slices, probably due to the fact that, contrary to the intestinal epithelium, the glucose transported by nervous tissue is rapidly utilized (Quastel 1965) and therefore it is impossible to record quantitative differences between the control and experimental brain cortex.

The disappearance of differences in O_2 consumption at a 30 mM concentration of glucose and alanine suggests that most probably in the cerebral cortex a competitive type of glucose transport inhibition takes place. The dependence of the alanine effect on the intact cell membranes and on the presence of sodium ions in the medium as well as the lack of sensitivity of membrane ATP-ase to alanine suggest that alanine influences glucose transport across the membrane. The direct influence of alanine on ion transport is in our opinion less probable. Nor was it found by Gilles-Bailieu and Schoffeniels (1967) who measured the fluxes of ions across the intestinal epithelium.

Alanine also inhibited aerobic glycolysis in stimulated tissue. Based on experiments with homogenates and slices with 5 mM potassium in the incubation medium, when alanine did not have any effect on lactate formation but reduced it in slices in a medium with 105 mM KCl, it seems probable that alanine does not inhibit the enzyme activity of glycolytic cycle and that the lower lactate formation in stimulated tissue in the presence of alanine is due to the lack of glucose supplied to the slices.

The decrease of metabolism in potassium-stimulated slices under the influence of L-α-alanine indicates that products of nervous tissue metabolism may also condition its activity and that in addition to the GABA shunt which is considered a process conditioning the inhibition in the nervous system (Jasper, Khan and Elliot 1965), there is also another way — the formation of α-alanine in tissue in the presence of elevated intracellular sodium chloride which by interfering with glucose transport can reduce the energy production needed for the functioning of the nervous system.

MORPHOLOGICAL AND METABOLIC CHANGES IN THE CEREBRAL CORTEX FOLLOWING TOPICAL APPLICATION OF KCl SOLUTIONS

KCl solutions, when applied to the surface of the cerebral cortex, cause in nerve cells a reversible reduction of gallocyanin bond to cellular structures (Ruščáková 1964a, b). In keeping with data reported in the literature (Hydén 1943, 1960, Einarson 1957, Danilova 1958), these findings were considered as evidence of a decrease in ribonucleoprotein structures in nerve cells under the influence of KCl. On the other hand, Cohen (1962) maintains that between the bond of gallocyanin and the RNA cell content which binds this dye no direct relationship exists; in nerve cells incubated *in vitro* in an atmosphere of O_2 or N_2 the bond of gallocyanin to cell structures was reduced, while the RNA content determined chemically remained unaltered. It was therefore assumed that the gallocyanin bond is conditioned not so much by the amount but rather by the shape and size of RNA molecules and the number of their functional groups binding the dye. In an effort to confirm the effect of KCl solutions on the nucleic acid content in the cerebral cortex further experiments were carried out. For the detection of nucleic acids the staining with methyl green-pyronin, which is supposed to be specific for nucleic acids (Brachet 1957), was used; the nucleic acid content of tissue was also determined spectrophotometrically (Goncharova and Broun 1964), according to the orcinol reaction (Ceriotti 1955) and phosphorus after mineralization of the nucleic acid extracts with $HClO_4$ according to Martin and Doty (1949).

Methyl green-positive material of the nucleus was found in the form of finely dispersed granules and a more intensely stained nucleolar satellite. Pyronin-positive material was found in the cytoplasm, nucleolus and nuclear membrane (figs. 27, 28).

The application of filter paper soaked in a 20 % solution of KCl on the cerebral cortex led in the cells of the layer I−IV to granulation and clumping of the methyl green-positive material and to a decrease of pyroninophilia (fig. 29). Changes in layers V−VI were similar but less marked, probably as a result of the dilution of the applied potassium during its penetration into deeper layers of the cortex. The cytoplasm of large pyramidal cells was paler; however, the appearance of the nucleus practically did not differ from controls (fig. 30). Restitution lasting 24 hr led in the large pyramidal cells to an increased pyroninophilia of the cytoplasm and perinuclear zone as well as of the nuclear contents (fig. 31). In the upper layers the main part of nerve cells returned to their initial appearance, but some of them did not manifest any signs of restitution (fig. 32). On the non-nerve cells no changes were found under the light microscope.

Substructural changes induced by 30 min application of a 20 % solution of potassium to the exposed cerebral cortex were manifested in the nerve cells by rarefaction of the ribosomal component and a partial loss of profiles of the endoplasmic reticulum (figs 33, 34). The less compact appearance of mitochondria was caused by dilatation of the cristae and reduced density of the mitochondrial matrix. After 4 hr the appearance of the nerve cells practically returned to normal. In the apical portions of the pyramidal cells the enhanced formation of parallely formed profiles of

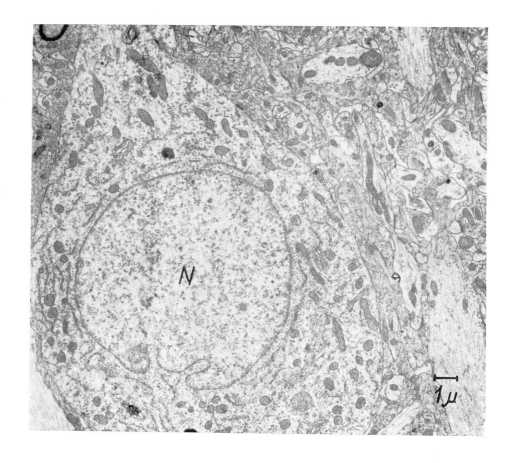

Fig. 33. Nerve cell of control cortex. N — nucleus.

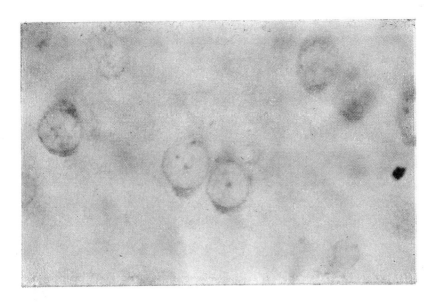

Fig. 27. Control layer III. Methyl green-pyronin.

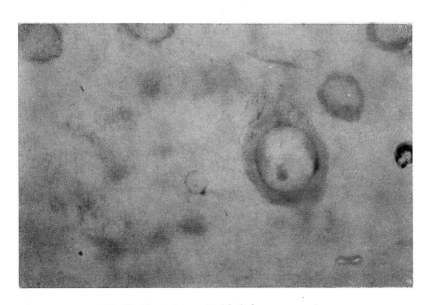

Fig 28. Control layer V. Methyl green-pyronin.

Erratum

Fig. 29 was changed by mistake with fig. 32.

Erratum

Fig. 29 was changed by mistake with fig. 12.

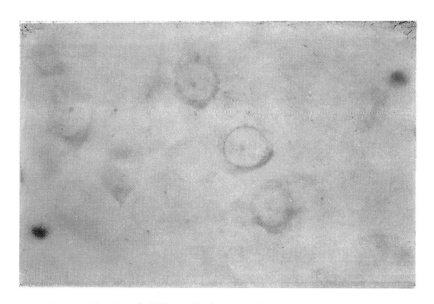

Fig. 29. After 30 min KCl application, layer III. Methyl green-pyronin.

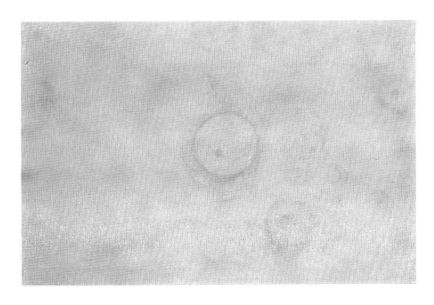

Fig. 30. After 30 min KCl application, layer V. Methyl green-pyronin.

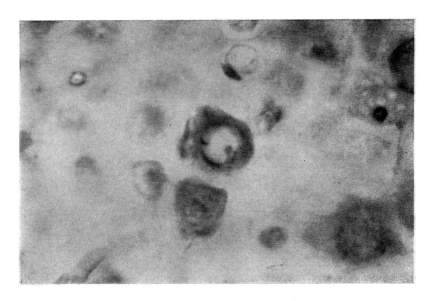

Fig. 31. After 30 min KCl application 24 hr recovery period, layer V. Methyl green-pyronin.

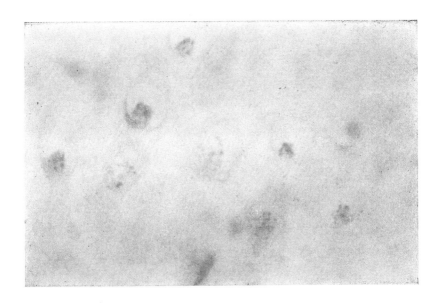

Fig. 32. After 30 min KCl application 24 hr recovery period, layer III. Methyl green-pyronin.

Fig. 29

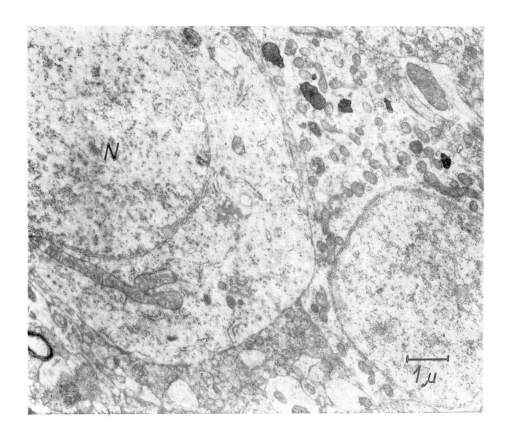

Fig. 34. Nerve cell following 30 min KCl application. N — nucleus of the nerve cell.

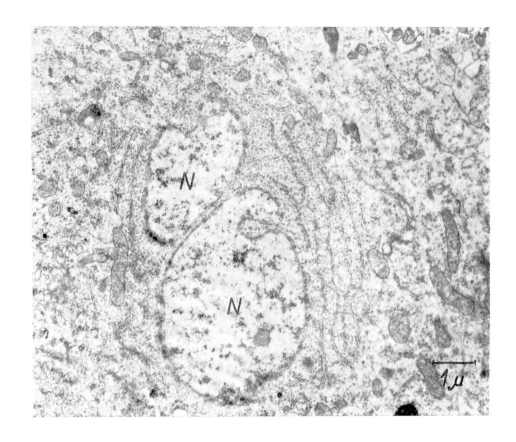

Fig. 35. Nerve cell following 30 min KCl application and 24 hr restitution period. N — nucleus.

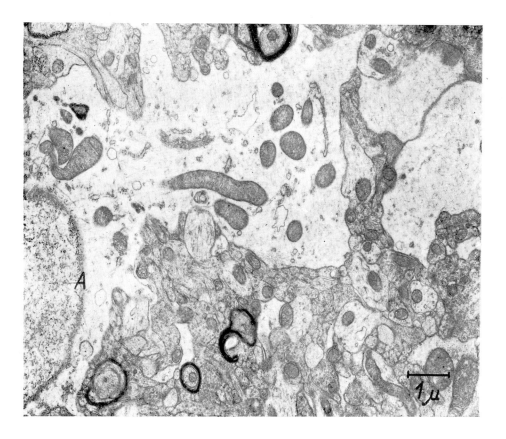

Fig. 36. Astroglial cell (A) following 30 min KCl application.

endoplasmic reticulum was frequently observed (fig. 35). This finding can be designed as structural equivalent of so-called Altmann's nuclear caps and is assumed to be the morphological manifestation of an enhanced physiological activity of the nerve cell.

The astroglia responds markedly to the direct action of potassium ions. Immediately after 30 min application of the KCl solution a reactive intracellular edema developed (fig. 36). After 24 hr the edematous changes recede partly but the number of mitochondria strikingly increases (figs. 37). They are smaller than in the intact cells and display different signs of alteration of the membranes and cristae. Concurrently with these changes the amount of carbohydrates in the astrocytic cytoplasm increased (figs 38, 39). There seems to be an inverse relationship between the amount of glycogen granules and the increase in the number of mitochondria. As the small mitochondria are usually arranged in the perinuclear

129

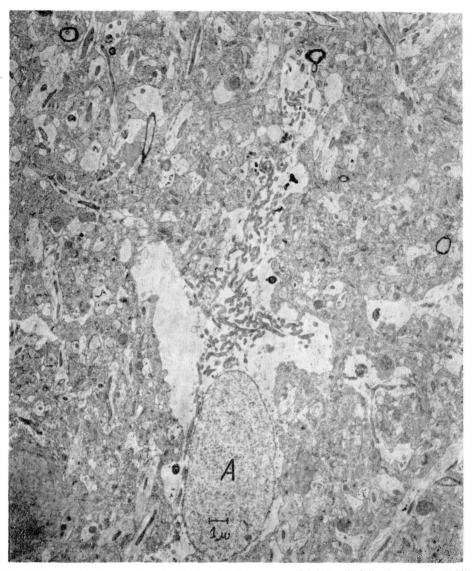

Fig. 37. Increase in the number of mitochondria in an astroglial (A) cell following 30 min KCll application and 24 hr restitution period.

zone or in the proximal part of the astrocytic processes, glycogen cumulate mainly in the pericapillary processes of the astrocytes, the so-called end-feets, which adhere closely to the vascular wall. The described changes which were particularly marked 24 hr after KCl application gradually receded and in the perinuclear area of the glial cytoplasm filamentous material began to increase. The number of mitochondria became reduced except for small groups deposited near the nucleus (figs 40, 41).

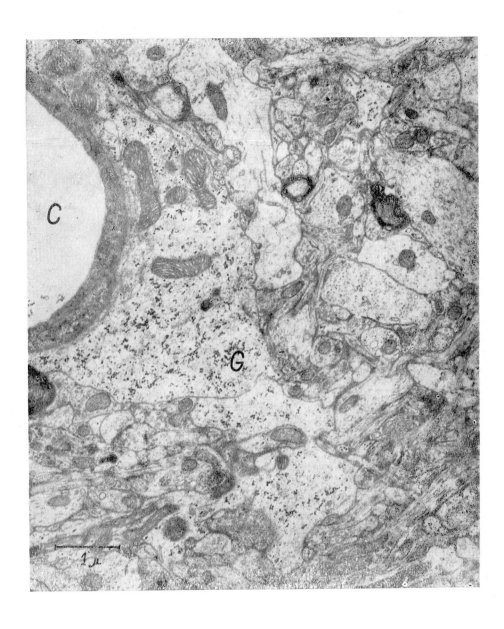

Figs 38, 39. Deposition of glycogen (G) in astroglial cells following 30 min KCl application and 24 hr restitution period. C — capillary.

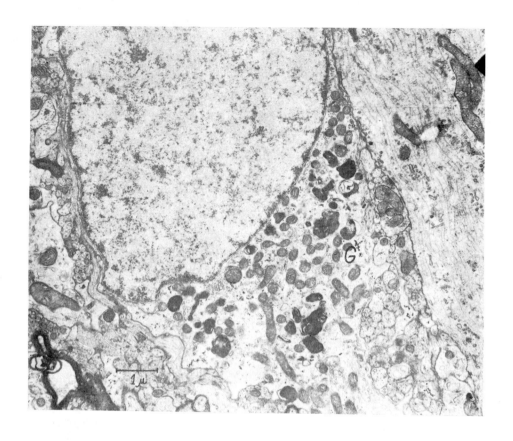

Fig. 39.

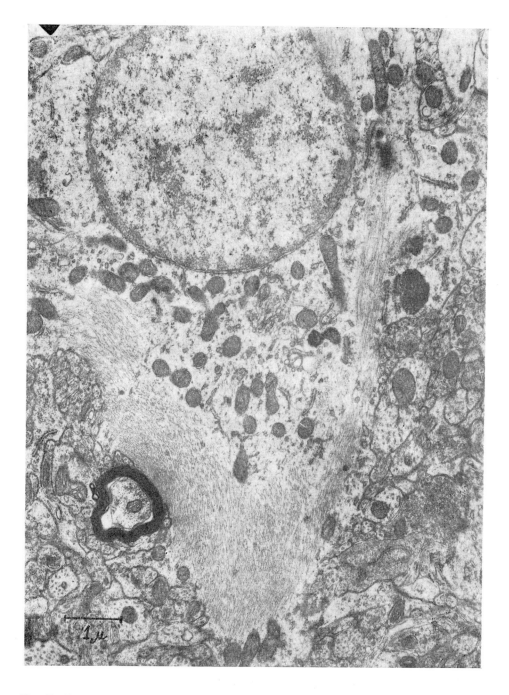

Figs 40, 41. Formation of gliofilaments in astroglial cells following 30 min KCl application **and** 96 hr restitution period.

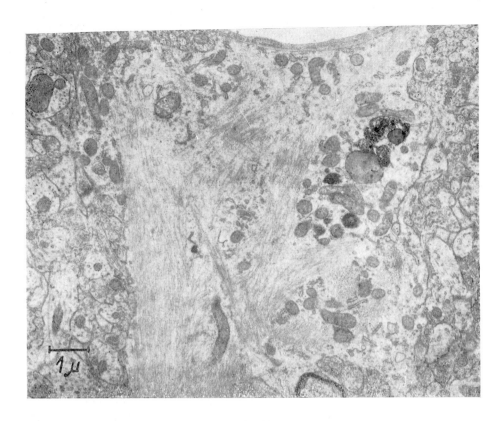

Fig. 41.

As can be seen from the results of chemical analyses (table 33), no differences in the RNA and DNA content between the right and left hemisphere of the same animal were observed. Because 30 min application of a 20 % solution of KCl led to a decrease in the dry matter from an average of 19.93 ± 0.14 g/100 g wet wt to 18.88 ± 0.13 g/100 g wet wt ($n = 9$, $P < 0.01$), all results were calculated on a dry weight basis. The effect of applied KCl was manifested in a decrease in RNA determined by the above described three methods, while the DNA content remained unaltered. The 24 hr restitution led to a slight but insignificant rise in RNA without changes in DNA. Evidence of the fact that potassium had an influence on the RNA content of tissue was provided even more markedly by the difference in its content when comparing groups after 30 min exposure to KCl and the group after 24 hr restitution. In the latter an increase by as much as 13 % was recorded.

Staining with methyl green-pyronin, which stain RNA and DNA selectively (Brachet 1957), gave similar results as staining with gallocyanin (Ruščáková 1964a), when under the influence of KCl a reduced pyroninophilia of nerve cells was observed. This finding can be considered as further evidence of a diminution of RNA, as it has

134

Table 33

	I		II		III		IV	
	C	E	C	E	C	E	C	E
1	300 ± 8	299 ± 10.5	77.5 ± 0.1	77 ± 0.13	90 ± 0.9	88.4 ± 1	41.35 ± 0.06	41.15 ± 0.03
		n. s.		n. s.		n. s.		n. s.
2	300 ± 5.3	281 ± 6.7	78.3 ± 0.59	74 ± 1	94 ± 1.9	80 ± 2	40.4 ± 0.08	40 ± 0.05
		P < 0.05		P < 0.01		P < 0.01		n. s.
3	297 ± 6	316 ± 5.8	79.5 ± 0.72	84.5 ± 2.6	92 ± 1.2	96.6 ± 2.9	40.7 ± 0.03	40.9 ± 0.05
		P < 0.05		n. s.		n. s.		n. s.

RNA ribose (I) and phosphorus estimated by means of spectrophotometric (II) and colorimetric (III) methods and DNA phosphorus (IV) in control (C) and experimental (E) rat brain cortex in mg as M ± S. E. M./100 g dry wt. 1 — no stimulus, 2 — following 30 min KCl application, 3 — 24 hr restitution after 30 min KCl application. Mean values of 12 experiments. n. s. — differences statistically not significant.

been proved that there exists a direct relationship between the RNA content of the cell estimated by cytospectrophotometry and the bond of basic dyes to cell structures (Landström et al. 1941, Danilova 1958). Finally also the electron microscopic findings revealed a drop in ribosomes, the main constituent of which is RNA, in neurons exposed to the action of KCl. A decrease in RNA in nerve cells was also found by other authors during exhaustive stimulation (Hamberger and Hydén 1949, Kulenkampf 1951, Hydén 1960) or during ischemia of the brain (Danilova 1958, Pevzner 1963).

Twenty-four hours after application of KCl an increased pyroninophilia was observed, in particular in the perinuclear zone of nerve cells. Brattgård, Edström and Hydén (1957) consider this phenomenon a result of redistribution of RNA polymers inside the cell without quantitative changes. We assume, however, that the more intense staining with pyronin was conditioned also by a rise in neuronal RNA, although we do not rule out that the altered RNA distribution contributed to the enhanced staining of the cytoplasm surrounding the nucleus, as could be shown also by the results of chemical analyses.

In keeping with results of chemical analyses, we did not observe any changes in the DNA content, except for the shrinkage of methyl green-positive material. Similar findings were described by Haymaker and Strughold (1957) in cells of the cerebral cortex after hypoxia. The reason for these findings is so far obscure, but the increase water content in the tissue and the fixation technique could, no doubt, play an important role.

The slight decrease in RNA obtained by chemical methods and, on the other hand, the marked differences in the histochemical picture can be explained by the fact that neurons, which were affected most by the action of KCl, represent only about 20 % of the total cell population of rat brain cortex and only one-half of the total volume of the tissue (Nurnberger 1958, Waelsch 1959). Since, however, in data of chemical analyses the results were related to tissue as a whole, the slight drop in RNA is understandable.

A decrease in RNA in nervous tissue after its stimulation is reported by several authors. Geiger (1958) found a lowered level of RNA in the sensory motor area in cats stimulated afferently via the plexus brachialis or directly by electrical current. Chitre, Chopra and Talwar (1964) described a reduced RNA level in the cortex of rats after Metrazol convulsions; particularly remarkable was their finding that except nervous tissue no other organ responded to Metrazol-induced convulsions by a decrease in RNA.

The reason for the decreased RNA content after application of potassium is most probably its utilization in energy processes as well as its reduced resynthesis (Křivánek 1959, Chitre, Chopra and Talwar 1964). Because potassium increased energy needs for processes associated with active ion transport (Grenell 1959, Gonda and Quastel 1962, Hertz and Schou 1962, Ruščák and Whittam 1967 and others), less energy was available for so-called plastic processes, such as protein and nucleic acid synthesis and thus the final result was a reduced RNA content. Also the alteration of the cell nuclei which are the site of RNA synthesis (Bondy 1966) might be the reason for a lower RNA level in the cortex under the direct influence of KCl.

Also remarkable was the finding that $2-4$ hr of exposure to KCl did not alter the RNA level more than 30 min exposure. It seems probable therefore that there is in the CNS only one RNA fraction which responds by a decrease to potassium stimulation.

The insignificant increase in the RNA content after 24 hr can be explained by the great variability of the reaction in different cell layers (Ruščáková 1964b). If we compare, however, the RNA values after 30 min and 24 hr application of KCl, the higher production of RNA in the potassium-stimulated cortex is obvious. This phenomenon reminds one of the so-called supercompensation in restitution processes well-known from the chemistry of striated muscle (Yakovlev 1958).

In O_2 consumption and lactic acid formation, despite marked morphological changes of nerve cells, no differences were found as compared with intact tissue, not even when KCl acted for as long as 4 hr and the medium contained 5 or 105 mM external K^+ resp. Only after 24 hr restitution a slight decrease in the O_2 consumption and glycolysis was found which was more marked when the metabolism of the slices was stimulated by raising the level of external potassium in the me-

Table 34

		I	II	III	IV
A	O_2	92 ± 3.2	95 ± 1.8	86 ± 2.7	94 ± 3.4
	LA	14.4 ± 1.8	17 ± 2	12.7 ± 2.2	16.2 ± 2.1
B	O_2	144 + 3.6	147 ± 3.1	128 ± 1.2	150 ± 4.2
	LA	34 ± 2.5	36.6 ± 2.7	28.2 ± 2.7	38 ± 3.6

Oxygen consumption (O_2) and lactic acid (LA) formation in rat brain cortex slices in μmoles as M ± S. E. M./g wet wt/hr. I — control experiments, II — 30 min application of 3 M KCl, III — 24 hr after KCl application, IV — 96 hr after KCl application. Mean values of 6 measurements. A — 5 mM potassium in the medium, B — 105 mM potassium in the medium.

dium to 105 mM. This decrease was reversible; already four days after the application of KCl no differences were observed between the control and experimental hemispheres (table 34). The reason for the decrease in O_2 consumption is the damage or disappearance of a part of the neurons in the surface layers of the brain cortex (Ruščáková 1964b), which have, as demonstrated in chapter 2, an O_2 consumption of higher order than non-nerve cells. In the astroglia of the upper layers of the cortex reactive changes occurred simultaneously and glycogen was deposited (figs 38, 39). These results again confirm the above given view that the decreased brain metabolism as a result of the elimination or structural alteration of neurons is the reason for glycogen deposition in the astroglia.

INFLUENCE OF EEG DEPRESSION ON INCORPORATION OF ^{35}S METHIONINE INTO PROTEINS OF THE CEREBRAL CORTEX IN RATS IN SITU

As mentioned above, during EEG depression depolarization as well as a decrease in electrical activity of the nervous tissue are observed (Brinley, Kandel and Marshall 1960, Křivánek and Bureš 1960). Because the reduced neuronal activity caused by various drugs (Palladin, Belik and Krachko 1957, Nechaeva 1957, Richter 1959) as well as the increase in external potassium in the incubation medium above values of the extracellular fluid in experiments with brain slices *in vitro* (Lindau, Quastel and Sved 1957, Bassi and Bernelli 1960, Folbergrová 1961) have shown that under these conditions the renewal of brain proteins investigated by means of labelled amino acids is reduced, we decided to investigate by means of ^{35}S methionine to what extent EEG depression will affect the turnover of the cortical proteins, as during EEG depression both above-mentioned phenomena appear simultaneously, i. e. the temporarily reduced neuronal activity and the rise of extracellular potassium.

In experiments on white rats EEG depression was elicited by applying filter paper soaked in 3 M KCl to the brain cortex surface. Closely before applying KCl to the animals i. p. ^{35}S methionine, (10,000 imp. /min/ g body weight) was administered. After decapitation of the animals the cortex was removed on ice; in the proteins of the cortex the activity by means of a G. M. tube in an infinitely thick layer was determined. The statistical evaluation of the results was made by the pair variation of the *t*-test and as controls the contralateral hemispheres of the same animal were taken.

It was found that already 30 min after the administration of ^{35}S methionine and simultaneous application of KCl to the cortex the specific activity in the experimental hemispheres decreased. When KCl was applied for 30 min and ^{35}S methionine administered simultaneously, but after 30 min application the KCl solution was washed off and the animals still survived 90 min, even under these conditions in the experimental hemisphere a decrease in specific activity of proteins was observed. A decrease in specific activity in the depressed cortex was found also if ^{35}S methionine was administered to the animals only at the end of the action of 3 M KCl. These experiments showed that the fall in specific activity was not caused by a direct action of the potassium applied to the cortex because that part of the cortex directly exposed to the action of KCl was removed. The reduced activity was not due to a possible so-called "injury stress" caused by trepanation or by the application of indifferent solutions to the cortex, as we found in our experiments that 90 min after 30 min exposure to physiological saline practically no differences in the specific activity of cortical proteins were found.

Statistically significant differences in specific activity of proteins between the control hemisphere and the hemisphere under the influence of EEG depression disappeared 24 hr after 30 min exposure to KCl (for summarized results see table 35).

These results demonstrated that the EEG depression decreased the incorporation of ^{35}S methionine into cortical proteins, similarly as reported in experiments *in vitro* where the potassium concentration of the incubation medium was increased (Lindau, Quastel and Sved 1957, Bassi and Bernelli 1960, Folbergrová 1961). This seems to indicate that between the experiments with a raised K^+ level *in vitro* and our results a certain analogy exists, as it is known that during the negative phase of the depression wave potassium is liberated from nervous elements into the extracellular space in amounts exceeding the threshold concentration needed for evoking the EEG depression (Křivánek and Bureš 1960, Brinley, Kandel and Marshall 1960). A certain role in the reduction of protein renewal under the influence of EEG depression elicited in our experiments by K^+ ions may be conditioned probably by submicroscopic changes in microsomal structures of nervous elements associated with the Nissl substance. This statement is based on our own experiments in which following local application of KCl solutions to the cortex of rats already at relatively low concentrations changes in the histological picture of nerve cells, among others also a diminution of the Nissl substance and ribosomal structures, were observed. When during EEG depression the extracellular potassium is increased it is possible that the rise in potassium causes a decrease or molecular changes in the microsomal fraction of nervous elements; thus a decrease in the specific activity of cortical proteins could be influenced by molecular changes of structures which participate directly in the incorporation of labelled amino acids into proteins (Clouet and Richter 1957, Palladin, Belik and Krachko 1959).

The fact that a decrease in specific activity of cortical proteins was found also after the action of KCl had ceased would suggest the important participation of the microsomal fraction in this process because histological investigations showed a very slow restitution of the Nissl bodies after KCl ceased to act (Ruščáková 1964b). The probability of this hypothesis is confirmed also by the experiments of Křivánek (1959), who found under the influence of EEG depression a decrease in the specific activity of RNA, the main component of Nissl substance, in the brain of rats after the administration of ^{32}P. This provides evidence of the close relationship between protein and nucleic acid metabolism in cellular structures responsible for protein synthesis.

It is possible that the decreased turnover of cortical proteins as a result of EEG depression is conditioned also by the depletion of energy reserves of high energy phosphates in nervous tissue, the latter being essential for protein synthesis. The decrease in high energy phosphates may be due to the raised extracellular potassium during depression waves and successive higher energy needs for the active ion transport. This possibility is suggested by our previous experiments (Zachar and Ruščák 1958) as well as by some data reported in the literature on experiments *in vitro* in which a reduced phosphorus turnover and a decrease in high energy phosphates in nervous tissue were observed, when there was excess of K^+ ions in the medium, despite the fact that the O_2 and substrate consumption was increased (Abood 1956, Fonyó et al. 1958.)

We cannot even rule out the fact that the inactivity of nerve cells in the course of the depression wave contributes to a decreased ^{35}S methionine incorporation into

142

Table 35

	I		II		III		IV		V	
	C	E	C	E	C	E	C	E	C	E
	100 ± 0.9	97 ± 1	44.6 ± 2.8	37.6 ± 2.5	114.9 ± 4.4	88 ± 3	83.8 ± 5.5	65.7 ± 4.3	164.2 ± 4.6	151.4 ± 12.9
		$n = 6$		$n = 6$		$n = 6$		$n = 9$		$n = 9$
		n.s.		$P < 0.05$		$P < 0.01$		$P < 0.05$		n.s.

Specific activity of the proteins of rat brain cortex (counts/min/10 mg protein) as arithmetical mean ± S. E. M. following subcutaneous injection of ^{35}S methionine (10,000 imp./g weight) : I — 30 min 0.9 % NaCl application and 90 min restitution, II — 30 min 3 M KCl application, III — 30 min 3 M KCl application and 90 min restitution, IV — 30 min 3 M KCl application, then KCl washed off, ^{35}S methionine administered and cortex taken after 120, min, V — 30 min 3 M KCl application and 24 hr restitution. C — control hemisphere, E — experimental hemisphere. n.s. — differences statistically not significant.

proteins, as it is known that the decrease in activity of nervous elements caused either by drugs (Palladin, Belik and Krachko 1957, Nechaeva 1957, Richter 1959) or by another physiological diminution of activity of the CNS (Belik 1963) slows down the turnover of labelled amino acids in brain proteins. Finally a lower level of ^{35}S methionine in the extracellular fluid in the experimental cortex and the resulting lower labelling of cortical proteins cannot be excluded, although in our experiments an increased activity in the soluble fraction was found; this fact could, however, not be ascribed to the actual amount of ^{35}S methionine present in the tissue but to a higher blood volume with high activity present in the depressed hemispheres (Burešová 1957).

It seems that the decrease in ^{35}S methionine incorporation during EEG depression may be influenced by several factors which in their mutual interaction probably condition the reduced turnover of cortical proteins.

SUMMARY

In the present publication the authors summarize their investigations on the metabolism of the CNS *in vitro* and *in situ* in relation to potassium and sodium ion movements and confront their own findings with data reported in the literature. From their work the following conclusions emerge:

1. As compared with neurons non-nerve cells of the cerebral cortex *in vitro* have an O_2 consumption of lower order. About two-thirds of the total O_2 consumption is used for the production of energy associated with active ion transport.

2. Damage of the neuron or its elimination from the functional unit glia-neuron leads to deposition of glycogen in the astroglia.

3. The uptake of potassium by brain slices is conditioned by the presence of nerve cells, similarly as increased O_2 consumption induced by extra potassium. The ratio Ca^{++}/K^+ is an important factor regulating the metabolism of nervous tissue *in vitro*. The elimination of Ca^{++} from a medium containing 5 mM K^+ or addition of Ca^{++} to a medium containing 105 mM K^+ enhances the metabolism of cerebral cortex slices, in spite of the fact that Ca^{++} has no influence on $Na^+ + K^+$-dependent ATP-ase activity. The rise in calcium above the so-called physiological value leads also in stimulated tissue to a decrease in O_2 consumption. Ouabain inhibits the metabolism when the K^+ level of the medium is high, similarly as in a Ca^{++}-free medium, while it has a stimulating effect in the presence of calcium and low potassium, although at the same time it inhibits active ion transport. The stimulating effect of calcium was observed already at a concentration of 0.1 mM. The omission of Ca^{++} or addition of extra 100 mM K^+ increases aerobic glycolysis. Oligomycin reduces the accumulation of tissue potassium; however, its influence on ion transport is not manifested by inhibition of the activity of transport ATP-ase but by inhibition of ATP energy production in the electron transport system. Oligomycin stimulates the aerobic and anaerobic lactic acid production. The inhibitory metabolic effect of ouabain and oligomycin are conditioned by the presence of sodium in the medium.

4. Depolarization of the cerebral cortex associated with EEG depression during bilateral ligature of the carotid arteries leads in experimental animals to a decrease in glycogen and glucose, to a rise in lactic and citric acids, while the α-keto acid levels remain unaltered. The restitution of the initial state is possible only after repeated renewal of the blood supply to the brain via the carotid arteries.

5. The increased lactic acid production during stimulation of nervous tissue *in vitro* as well as *in situ* is conditioned by the presence of nerve cells.

6. It has been found that the lactic acid production takes place also in the crude mitochondrial fraction isolated from the hemispheres of rats. A significantly lower production of lactate from glucose-1-phosphate as compared with glucose and fructose-1,6-diphosphate suggests that the main source for the formation of lactic acid in the CNS is glucose and not glycogen. Purified mitochondria prepared by centrifuging through a sucrose density gradient practically lost their glycolytic properties. This finding proved that as regards glycolysis there was no difference between mito-

chondria of the CNS and other organs. In structures containing transport ATP-ase (in the sub-fraction of membranes and nerve endings) the production of lactic acid is stimulated by sodium ions and inhibited by ouabain in the medium. This fact provides evidence of the participation of Na^+ and K^+-dependent ATP-ase in the regulation of glycolysis in the CNS.

7. Depolarization of the cerebral cortex during EEG depression when the carotid arteries were ligated was accompanied by a decrease in aspartic acid, glutamic acid and glutamine and a rise in γ-aminobutyric acid and α-alanine. The reversibility of these changes is conditioned by the restitution of blood supply through the carotid arteries.

8. The GABA shunt in the CNS is bound to nerve cells.

9. The formation of α-alanine in the cortex is conditioned by the utilization of glutamic acid in oxidative processes. Under aerobic conditions sodium stimulated α-alanine formation from glutamic and pyruvic acid; under anaerobic conditions sodium also stimulated α-alanine formation. Stimulation of α-alanine production by sodium under aerobic conditions does not depend on the activity of $Na^+ + K^+ + Mg^{++}$-dependent ATP-ase, as in the presence of ouabain we did not observe any effect on α-alanine formation. Ouabain, however, reduced the production of aspartic acid and stimulated the formation of γ-aminobutyric acid.

The enzymes producing α-alanine were found in mitochondria and in the soluble fraction; no differences in specific activity were observed between gray and white matter of the CNS. The soluble enzyme is uninfluenced while the mitochondrial one is inhibited in the presence of Cl^- ions. Chloride inhibition begins at 80 mM, half-maximal effect is at 100 mM and maximal inhibitory effect was reached at 150 mM Cl^- concentration. KCl is more effective than NaCl. pH optimum of the soluble enzyme is 7.5-8 while that of mitochondrial one has a plateau between 7.5-9. Mitochondrial enzyme is three times more inhibited in the presence of maleic acid than the soluble one. p-Chloromercuribenzoate inactivates both enzymes to the same extent. Mitochondrial enzyme can be solubilized by means of sonification without any change of its properties.

10. L-α-alanine inhibited the metabolism of cerebral cortex slices stimulated by addition of 105 mM potassium to the medium. Because the inhibitory effect was not observed when pyruvate was used as substrate and disappeared when the glucose concentration reached the α-alanine level in the medium, it is assumed that L-α-alanine inhibits the metabolism of nerve tissue by reducing competitively the glucose transport to the cells. Since it has no effect on the activity of membrane ATP-ase, it seems improbable that α-alanine has any direct effect on the metabolism via the membrane ATP-ase. It is ineffective in homogenates and its effect depends on the presence of sodium in the medium.

11. Potassium ions when applied to the surface of the cerebral cortex cause a de-

148

crease in RNA in nerve cells, which could be detected by histochemical, electronoptical and chemical methods.

12. Depolarization of the cerebral cortex *in situ* is associated similarly as *in vitro* by a reduced turnover rate of proteins.

Bratislava, March 1968.

REFERENCES

Abood L. G., Chemical and energetic changes during nerve conduction and muscle activity. XX International physiological congress, Abstr. of Communications p. 9, Brussels 1956.

Abood L. G., Brunngraber E. and Taylor M., Glycolytic and oxidative phosphorylative studies with intact and disrupted rat brain mitochondria. J. biol. Chem. 234 : 1307, 1959.

Adler M. and Hollander F., Determination of reducing sugars in the presence of amino acids and polypeptides. Feder. Proc. 12 : 166, 1953.

Albers R. W., Gamma-aminobutyric acid. In: The Neurochemistry of Nucleotides and Amino Acids. John Wiley and Sons Inc., New York-London 1960, p. 146.

Albers R. W. and Brady R. O., The distribution of glutamic decarboxylase in the nervous system of the Rhesus monkey. J. biol. Chem. 234 : 926, 1959.

Albers R. W. and Salvador R. A., Succinic semialdehyde oxidation by a soluble dehydrogenase from brain. Science 128 : 359, 1958.

Aldridge W. N., Liver and brain mitochondria. Biochem. J. 67 : 423, 1957.

Alexandrovskaya M. M., Sosudistyje izmeneniya v mozgu pri razlichnykh patologicheskikh sostoyaniyakh. Medgiz, Moscow 1955.

Ashford Ch. A. and Dixon K. C., The effect of potassium on the glucolysis of brain tissue with reference to the Pasteur effect. Biochem. J. 29 : 157, 1935.

Awapara J., The influence of fluoracetate on the concentration of free amino acids in rat organs. J. biol. Chem. 197 : 695, 1952.

Awapara J., Landua A. J., Fuerst R. and Seale B., Free γ-aminobutyric acid in brain. J. biol. Chem. 187 : 35, 1950.

Awapara J. and Seale B., Distribution of transaminases in rat organs. J. biol. Chem. 194 : 497, 1952.

Bachelard H. S., Cerebral cortex hexokinase. Biochem. J. 102 : 21P, 1966.

Bain J. A. and Pollock G. H., Normal and seizure levels of lactate, pyruvate and acid soluble phosphates in the cerebellum and cerebrum. Proc. Soc. exp. Biol. Med. 71 : 495, 1949.

Bain J. A., Pollock G. H. and Stein S. N., Lactate, pyruvate and acid soluble phosphates in monkey brains treated with carbon dioxide and electric shock. Proc. Soc. exp. Biol. Med. 71 : 497, 1949.

Baker P. F., Phosphorus metabolism of intact crab nerve and its relation to the active transport of ions. J. Physiol. 180 : 383, 1965.

Baker P. F. and Connally C. M., Some properties of the external activation site of the sodium pump in crab nerve. J. Physiol. 185 : 270, 1966.

Balázs R., The point of the aerobic inhibition of glycolytic activity associated with brain mitochondria. Biochem. J. 72 : 561, 1959.

Balázs R., Control of glutamate metabolism. The effect of pyruvate. J. Neurochem. 12 : 63, 1965.

Balázs R. and Lagnado J. R., Glycolytic activity associated with rat brain mitochondria. J. Neurochem. 5 : 1, 1959.

Balázs R. and Richter D., The Pasteur effect in brain mitochondria. Biochem. J. 68 : 59, 1959.

Balzer H., Holtz P. and Palm D., Reserpin und γ-Aminobuttersäuregehalt des Gehirns. Experientia 17 : 38, 1961.

Barker S. B. and Summerson W. H., The colorimetric determination of lactic acid in biological material. J. biol. Chem. 138 : 535, 1941.

Barr M. L. and Bertram E. G., The behaviour of nuclear structures during depletion and restoration of Nissl material in motor neurons. A. Anat. (London) 85 : 171, 1951.

Basford R. E., Stahl W. L., Beattie D. S., Sloan H. R., Smith J. C. and Napolitano L. M., Enzymic properties of brain mitochondria. In: Morphological and Biochemical Correlates of Neural Activity. Ed. by M. M. Cohen and R. S. Snider, Harper and Row, New York 1964, p. 192.

153

Bassi M. and Bernelli Zazzera A., Effects of potassium ions on brain respiration and amino acid incorporation into brain proteins in vitro. Experientia 16 : 430, 1960.

Baxter C. F. and Roberts E., γ-Aminobutyric acid α-ketoglutaric acid transaminase in brain. Feder. Proc. 17 : 187, 1958.

Baxter C. F. and Roberts E., Elevation of γ-aminobutyric acid in rat brain with hydroxylamine. Proc. Soc. exp. Biol. Med. 101 : 811, 1959.

Baxter C. F. and Roberts E., Gamma-aminobutyric acid and cerebral metabolism. In: The Neuro-chemistry of Nucleotides and Amino Acids. John Wiley and Sons Inc., New York-London 1960, p. 127.

Baxter C. F., Roberts E. and Eidelberg E., γ-Aminobutyric acid and seizure susceptibility in areas of normal brain cortex. J. Neurochem. 5 : 203, 1960.

Beattie D. S., Sloan H. R. and Basford R. E., Relationship between brain mitochondria and glycolysis. Feder. Proc. 21 : 154, 1962.

Beattie D. S., Sloan H. R. and Basford R. E., Brain mitochondria. II. The relationship of brain mitochondria to glycolysis. J. Cell Biol. 19 : 309, 1963.

Belik Ja. V., Intensivnost obnovleniya summarnykh belkov i belkov subkletochnykh frakciy tkani golovnogo mozga suslikov. Tretya vsesoyuznaiya konferentsiya po biokhimiyi nervnoy sistemy. Akad. Nauk ASSR, Erevan 1963, p. 39.

Beloff-Chain A., Catanzaro R., Chain E. B., Masi J. and Pocchiari F., Fate of uniformly labelled ^{14}C glucose in brain slices. Proc. Roy. Soc. B. 144 : 22, 1955.

Beloff-Chain A., Catanzaro R., Chain E. B., Longinotti L., Masi J. and Pocchiari F., The influence of glucose on acetate, alanine and pyruvate metabolism in rat cerebral cortical slices. Proc. Roy. Soc. B. 156 : 168, 1962.

Bessman B. C. and Lardy H. A., Influence of potassium and other alkali cations on respiration of mitochondria. J. biol. Chem. 197 : 457, 1953.

Bessman S. P., Rossen J. and Layne E. C., γ-Aminobutyric acid — glutamic acid transamination in brain. J. biol. Chem. 201 : 385, 1953.

Bilodeau F. and Elliot K. A. C., The influence of drugs and potassium on respiration and potassium accumulation by brain tissue. Canad. J. Biochem. Physiol. 41 : 779, 1963.

Birmingham M. K. and Elliot K. A. C., Effects of pH, bicarbonate and cofactors on the metabolism of brain suspensions. J. biol. Chem. 189 : 73, 1949.

Blass J. P., The simple monosubstituted guanidines of mammalian brain. Biochem. J. 77 : 484, 1960.

Blaustein M. P. and Goldman D. E., Competitive action of calcium and procaine on Lobster. Z. mikr. anat. Forsch. 49 : 534, 1941.

Blaustein M. P. and Goldman D. E., Competitive action of calcium and procaine on Lobster axon. J. Gen. Physiol. 49 : 1038, 1966.

Blond D. J., Kresack E. J. and Kosicki G. W., The effects of ions and freeze-thawing on supernatant and mitochondrial malate dehydrogenase. Canad. J. Biochem. Physiol. 45 : 641, 1957.

Blond D. M. and Whittam R., The regulation of kidney respiration by sodium and potassium ions. Biochem. J. 92 : 158, 1964.

Bolingbroke V. and Maizels M., Calcium ions and the permeability of human erythrocytes. J. Physiol. 149 : 563, 1959.

Bondareff W., The extracellular compartment of the cerebral cortex. Anat. Rec. 152 : 119, 1965.

Bondy S. C., The ribonucleic acid metabolism of the brain. J. Neurochem. 13 : 955, 1966.

Borst P. and Slater E. C., The oxidation of glutamate by rat-heart sarcosomes. Biochim. biophys. Acta 41 : 170, 1960.

Boxer G. E. and Dewlin T. M., Pathways of intracellular hydrogen transport. Science 134 : 1495, 1961.

Boxer G. E. and Shonk C. E., Mitochondrial triose phosphate isomerase. Biochim. biophys. Acta 37 : 191, 1960.

Brachet J., Biochemical Cytology. Acad. Press, New York 1957.

Bradford H. F. and Rose S. P. R., Ionic accumulation and membrane properties of enriched preparation of neurons and glia from mammalian cerebral cortex. J. Neurochem. 14 : 373, 1967.

Brattgård S. O., Edström J. E. and Hydén H., The chemical changes in regenerating neurons. J. Neurochem. 1 : 316, 1957.

Braunstein A. E., Transamination and the integrative function of the dicarboxylic acids in nitrogen metabolism. Adv. Prot. Chem. 3 : 1, 1947.

Braunstein A. E., Biokhimiya aminokislotnogo obmena. AN SSSR, Moscow 1949.

Braunstein A. E., Glavnye puti assimilatsyi a dissimilatsyi azota u zhivotnykh. Izd. AN SSSR, Moscow 1957.

Brinley F. J., Kandel E. R. and Marshall W. H., Potassium outflux from rabbit cortex during spreading depression. J. Neurophysiol. 23 : 246, 1960.

Brody T. M. and Bain J. A., A mitochondrial preparation from mammalian brain. J. biol. Chem. 195 : 685, 1952.

Bronovickaya Z. G. and Shapovalova N. S., Glukoza i glikogen mozga pri dejstviyi na zhivotnykh povyshennogo davleniya kisloroda. Ukr. biokh. Zh. 27 : 20, 1957.

Brunngraber E. G. and Abood L. G., Mitochondrial glycolysis of rat brain and its relationship to the remainder of cellular glycolysis. J. biol. Chem. 235 : 1847, 1960.

Brunngraber E. G., Aguilar G. and Occomy W. G., The intracellular distribution of glycolytic and tricarboxylic acid cycle enzymes in rat brain mitochondrial preparations. J. Neurochem. 10 : 433, 1963.

Bukin Ju. V., Vliyanie vvedeniya antagonistov vitamina B_6 na soderzhanie NH_3, glutamina, glutamovoy i γ-aminomaslyanoy kislot v mozgu krys. Ukr. biokh. Zh. 31 : 906, 1959.

Bunyatyan G. Ch., Novye dannye u roli gammaaminomaslyanoy kisloty. Dokl. Akad. Nauk SSSR 132 : 1431, 1960.

Bunyatyan H. Ch., The role of γ-aminobutyric acid in the metabolism of glutamic acid and glutamine in brain. J. Neurochem. 10 : 461, 1963.

Bureš J., Some metabolic aspects of Leão's spreading depression. J. Neurochem. 1 : 153, 1956.

Bureš J. and Burešová O., K otázce antagonismu iontů při šířící se depresi. Čs. fysiol. 5 : 174, 1956.

Bureš J. and Burešová O., Vliv elektrošoku a šířící se EEG deprese na přetrvání dočasných spojů. Čs. fysiol. 9 : 5, 1960.

Burešová O., Changes in cerebral circulation of rats during spreading EEG depression. Physiol. bohemoslov. 6 : 1, 1957.

du Buy H. G. and Hesselbach M. L., Carbohydrates and carbohydrate metabolite utilisation by enzyme systems of mouse brain and liver mitochondria. J. Histochem. Cytochem. 4 : 363, 1956.

Cacioppo F., Pandolfo L. and di Chiaria G., Transaminazione acido γ-aminobutyrrico-acido α-chetoglutarico in alcuni tessuti di ratto. Boll. Soc. ital. Biol. sperim. 35 : 465, 1959.

Carter S. H. and Stone W. E., Effect of convulsants on brain glycogen in the mouse. J. Neurochem. 7 : 16, 1961.

Caspersson T., Cell Growth and Cell Function. Norton, New York 1950.

Cavallini D. and Fontali N., Quantitative determination of keto acids by paper partition chromatography. Biochim. biophys. Acta 13 : 439, 1954.

Ceriotti G., Determination of nucleic acids in animal tissues. J. biol. Chem. 214 : 59, 1955.

Chain E. B., Cohen M. M. and Pocchiari F., Interrelationships of glucose, glutamate and aspartate metabolism in rat cerebral cortical slices. Proc. Roy. Soc. B. 156 : 163, 1962.

Chajkina B. I., Obmen frakciy glikogena golovnogo mozga pri rozlichnykh sostoyaniyakh organizma. In: Uglevody i uglevodniy obmen v zhivotnom i rastitelnom organizmakh. Izd. AN SSSR Moscow 1959.

Chappel J. B., Cohn M. and Greville G. D., The accumulation of bivalent ions by isolated mitochondria. In: Energy-Linked Functions of Mitochondria. Ed. by B. Chance, Acad. Press, New York 1963, p. 129.

Chitre V. S., Chopra S. P. and Talwar G. P., Changes in the ribonucleic acid content of the brain during experimentally induced convulsions. J. Neurochem. 11 : 439, 1964.

Clouet D. E. and Richter D., The incorporation of ^{35}S methionine into protein fractions of the brain. Biochem. J. 65 : 20P, 1957.

Cohen H. P., Phosphorylation coupled to glycolytic and oxidative metabolism in cerebral mitochondrial systems. Arch. Biochem. Biophys. 92 : 449, 1961.

Cohen M. M., The effect of anoxia on the chemistry and morphology of cerebral cortex slices in vitro. J. Neurochem. 9 : 337, 1962.

Cohen M. M. and Cohen H. P., The effect of glutamic acid on phosphorus metabolism in cerebral tissue preparations. J. Neurochem. 13 : 811, 1966.

Cohen M. M. and Hartmann J. F., Biochemical and ultrastructural correlates of cerebral cortex slices metabolizing in vitro. In: Morphological and Biochemical Correlates of Neural Activity. Ed. by M. M. Cohen and R. S. Snider, Harper and Row, New York 1964, p. 57.

Cohen M. M., Simon G. R., Berry J. F. and Chain E. B., Conversion of glutamic acid into aspartic acid in cerebral cortex slices. Biochem. J. 84 : 43P, 1962.

Cohen P. P., Transamination in pigeon breast muscle. Biochem. J. 33 : 147, 1939.

Cohen P. P. and Hekhuis L., Rate of transamination in normal tissues. J. biol. Chem. 140 : 711, 1940.

Coon M. J. and Robinson W. G., Amino acid metabolism. Ann. Rev. Biochem. 27 : 561, 1958.

Copenhaver J. H., McShan W. H. and Meyer R. K., The determination of glutamic dehydrogenase in tissue homogenate. J. biol. Chem. 183 : 73, 1950.

Coxon R. V., Liébecq C. and Peter R. A., The pyruvate oxidase system in brain and tricarboxylic acid cycle. Biochem. J. 45 : 320, 1949.

Cravioto R. O., Massieu G. and Izquierdo J. J., Free amino acids in rat brain during insulin shock. Proc. Soc. exp. Biol. Med. 78 : 856, 1951.

Cremer J. E., The actions of mitochondrial preparations on glycolysis. Biochim. biophys. Acta 41 : 155, 1960.

Curran P. F., Herrera F. C. and Flanigan W. J., The effect of calcium and antidiuretic hormone on sodium transport across frog skin. II. Sites and mechanism of action. J. gen. Physiol. 46 : 1011, 1963.

Damjanovich R., Fehér O., Halász P. and Mechler F., The effect of alpha-amino acids on ganglionic transmission. Acta physiol. Acad. Sci. Hung. 18 : 57, 1960.

Danilova O. D., Ultrafioletovaya mikroskopiya nekotorykh otdelov golovnogo mozga krolikov pri razlichnykh funkcionalnykh sostoyaniakh. Izv. Akad. Nauk SSSR, ser. biol. 23 : 161, 1958.

Davis B. D., Intermediates in amino acids biosynthesis. Adv. Enzymol. 16 : 247, 1955.

Dawson J. and Bone A., Water uptake by, and sodium and potassium content of brain slices. J. Neurochem. 12 : 167, 1965.

Dawson R. M. C., Studies on the glutamine and glutamic acid content of the rat brain during insulin hypoglycaemia. Biochem. J. 47 : 386, 1950.

Dawson R. M. C., Cerebral amino acids in fluoracetate poisoned anesthetized and hypoglycaemic rat. Biochim. biophys. Acta 11 : 548, 1955.

Dawson R. M. C. and Richter D., Effect of stimulation on the phosphate esters of the brain. Amer. J. Physiol. 160 : 203, 1950.

Deul D. H. and McIlwain H., Activation and inhibition of adenosinetriphosphatases of subcellular particles from the brain. J. Neurochem. 8 : 246, 1961.

Dickens F. and Greville G. D., The metabolism of normal and tumor tissues. XIII. Neutral salts effects. Biochem. J. 29 : 1468, 1935.

Dixon K. C., Action of potassium ions on brain metabolism. J. Physiol. 110 : 89, 1949.

Domonkos J. and Huszák I., Effect of hydrogen ion concentration on the carbohydrate metabolism of brain tissue. J. Neurochem. 4 : 238, 1959.

Dravid A. R. and Jílek L., Influence of stagnant hypoxia (oligaemia) on some free amino acids in rat brain during ontogeny. J. Neurochem. 12 : 837, 1965.

Duda P., Ruščák M. and Zachar J., Spreading cortical depression and the polarisation gradient of the cerebral cortex. Physiol. bohemoslov. 10 : 438, 1961.

Eidelberg E., Baxter C. F., Roberts E., Saldias C. A. and French J. D., Anticonvulsant properties of hydroxylamine and elevation of cerebral γ-aminobutyric acid in cats. Proc. Soc. exp. Biol. Med. 101 : 815, 1959.

Einarson L., Cytological aspects of nucleic acid metabolism. In: Metabolism of the Nervous System. Ed. D. Richter, Pergamon Press, London-New York-Paris-Los Angeles 1957, p. 403.

Elliot K. A. C., Brain tissue respiration and glycolysis. In: Neurochemistry. Ed. by K. A. C. Elliot, I. H. Page and J. H. Quastel, Ch. Thomas, Springfield, Ill. 1957, p. 53.

Elliot K. A. C., The chemical pathology of fluids and electrolytes. Brain swelling and fluid and electrolyte distribution. In: Chemical Pathology of the Nervous System. Ed. by J. Folch - Pi, Pergamon Press, New York-Oxford-London-Paris 1961, p. 277.

Elliot K. A. C., γ-Aminobutyric acid and other inhibitory substances. Brit. Med. J. 21 : 70, 1965.

Elliot K. A. C. and Bilodeau F., The influence of potassium on respiration and glycolysis by brain slices. Biochem. J. 84 : 42, 1962.

Elliot K. A. C. and Birmingham M. K., The effect of pH on the respiration of brain tissue; the pH of the tissue slices. J. biol. Chem. 177 : 51, 1949.

Elliot K. A. C. and van Gelder N. M., The state of Factor I in rat brain: the effects of metabolic conditions and drugs. J. Physiol. 153 : 423, 1960.

Elliot K. A. C. and Jasper H. H., Gamma-aminobutyric acid. Physiol. Rev. 39 : 383, 1959.

Elshove A. and van Rossum G. D. V., Net movements of sodium and potassium, and their relation to respiration in slices of rat liver incubated in vitro. J. Physiol. 168 : 531, 1963.

Epstein M. E. and O'Connor J. S., Respiration of single cortical neurons and of surrounding neuropile. J. Neurochem. 12 : 389, 1965.

Erbslöh F., Klärner P. and Brensmeier A., Die Milchsäureabgabe des menschlichen Gehirns. Pfl. Arch. 268 : 120, 1958.

v. Euler H., Adler E., Günther G. and Das N. B., Über den enzymatischen Abbau und Aufbau der Glutaminsäure. Z. physiol. Chemie 254 : 61, 1938.

Findlay M., Rossiter R. J. and Strickland K. P., Factors affecting the incorporation of radioactive phosphate into the pentosenucleic acids in brain slices. Biochem. J. 55 : 200, 1953.

Fischer F. G. and Dörfel H., Zur quantitativen Auswertung der Papierchromatogramme von Eiweiss-Hydrolysaten. Biochem. Z. 324 : 544, 1953.

Florey E., Physiological evidence for naturally occurring inhibitory substances. In: Inhibition in the Central Nervous System and Gamma-Aminobutyric Acid. Ed. by E. Roberts, Pergamon Press, Oxford-London, New York-Paris 1960, p. 72.

Folbergrová J., The effect of potassium and some other factors upon the incorporation of ^{35}S methionine into proteins of brain cortex slices. Physiol. bohemoslov. 10 : 130, 1961.

Folch-Pi J. and Le Baron F. N., Chemical composition of the mammalian nervous system. In: Metabolism of the Nervous System. Ed. by D. Richter, Pergamon Press, New York-London 1957, p. 67.

Fonnum F., The distribution of glutamate decarboxylase and aspartate transaminase in subcellular fractions of rat and guinea-pig brain. Biochem. J. 106 : 401, 1968.

Fonyó A., Kovách A. G. B., Makláry E., Leszkovszky G. and Mészáros J., The effect of potassium ions and glutamate on the incorporation of ^{32}P into nucleotides and phosphocreatine in brain slices. Acta physiol. Acad. Sci. Hung. 14 : 305, 1958.

Frankenhauser B. and Hodgkin A. L., The action of calcium on the electrical properties of squid axons. J. Physiol. 137 : 217, 1957.

Friede R., Die Bedeutung der Glia für den zentralen Kohlehydratstoffwechsel. Zbl. allg. Path. Anat. 92 : 65, 1954.

Friede R. L., The enzymatic response of astrocytes to various ions in vitro. J. Cell Biol. 20 : 5, 1964.

Friede R. L., Enzyme histochemistry of neuroglia. In: Biology of Neuroglia. Ed. by E. D. P. de Robertis and A. Carrea, Elsevier, Amsterdam 1965, p. 35.

Frontali N., Activity of glutamic acid decarboxylase in insect nerve tissue. Nature 191 : 178, 1961.

Gaevskaya M. C. and Nosova E. A., Osobennosti uglevodno-fosfornogo i azotistogo obmena mozga v usloviyakh glubokoy gipotermiyi. Tretya vsesoyuznaya konferentsiya po biokhimiyi nervnoy sistemy. AN ASSR, Erevan 1963, p. 421.

Gaitonde M. K., Richter D. and Vrba R., Utilisation of glucose in rat brain. Biochem. J. 84 : 105P, 1962.

Gallagher C. H., Judah J. D. and Rees K. R., Glucose oxidation by brain mitochondria. Biochem. J. 62 : 436, 1956.

Garfinkel D. and Hess B., Metabolic control mechanisms. VII. A detailed computer model of the glycolytic pathway in ascites cells. J. biol. Chem. 239 : 971, 1964.

Garland P. B., Randle P. J. and Newsholme E. A., Citrate as an intermediary in the inhibition of phosphofructokinase in rat heart muscle by fatty acids, ketone bodies, pyruvate, diabetes and starvation. Nature 200 : 169, 1963.

Geiger A., Correlation of brain metabolism and function by the use of a brain perfusion method in situ. Physiol. Rev. 38 : 1, 1958.

Geiger A., Domnas A., Kawakita J. and Nebel I., Incorporation of ^{14}C labelled glucose into various components of the brain during perfusion in situ. Feder. Proc. 17 : 52, 1958.

Geiger A., Horvath N. and Kawakita J., The incorporation of ^{14}C derived from glucose into the proteins of the brain cortex, at rest and during activity. J. Neurochem. 5 : 311, 1960.

Geiger A., Kawakita J. and Barkulis S. S., Major pathways of glucose utilisation in the brain perfusion experiments in vivo and in situ. J. Neurochem. 5 : 323, 1960.

Geiger A., Yamasaki S. and Lyons R., Changes in nitrogenous components of brain produced by stimulation of short duration. Amer. J. Physiol. 184 : 239, 1956.

van Gelder N. M., A comparison of γ-aminobutyric acid metabolism in rabbit and mouse nervous tissue. J. Neurochem. 12 : 239, 1965.

Gerard R. W., Metabolism and function in the nervous system. In: Neurochemistry. Ed. by K. A. C. Elliot, I. H. Page and J. H. Quastel, Ch. C. Thomas, Springfield, Ill. 1955, p. 458.

Gey K. F., The concentration of glucose in cat tissues. Biochem. J. 64 : 145, 1956.

Giacobini E., Metabolic relation between glia and neurons studied in single cells. In: Morphological and Biochemical Correlates of Neural Activity. Ed. by M. M. Cohen and R. S. Snider, Harper and Row, New York 1964, p. 177.

Giacobini E., Energy metabolism and ion transport studied in single neurons. Protoplasma 63 : 52, 1967.

Gibbs E. L., Lennox W. G., Nims L. F. and Gibbs F. A., Arterial and venous cerebral blood lactate. J. biol. Chem. 144 : 325, 1942.

Gilles-Bailieu M. and Schoffeniels E., Action of L-alanine on the fluxes of inorganic ions across the intestinal epithelium of the Greek tortoise. Life Sci. 6 : 1257, 1967.

Ginter E., Voľné aminokyseliny niektorých tkanív morčaťa. Biológia 13 : 700, 1958.

Glynn I. M., Activation of adenosinetriphosphatase activity in cell membrane by external potassium and internal sodium. J. Physiol. 160 : 18P, 1962.

Glynn I. M., Transport ATP-ase in electric organ. The relation between ion transport and oxidative phosphorylation. J. Physiol. 169 : 452, 1963.

Goncharova V. P. and Broun R. G., On the quantitative determination of nucleic acids in brain tissue. Ukr. biokh. Zh. 36 : 131, 1964.

Gonda O. and Quastel J. H., Effects of ouabain on cerebral metabolism and transport mechanisms in vitro. Biochem. J. 84 : 394, 1962.

Grafstein B., Mechanism of spreading cortical depression. J. Neurophysiol. 19 : 155, 1956.

Greenberg D. M., Amino Acids and Proteins. Ch. C. Thomas, Springfield, Ill. 1951.

Grenell R. G., Some molecular considerations in cerebral drug responses. In: Biochemistry of the Central Nervous System. Ed. by F. Bruecke, Pergamon Press, London-New York-Paris-Los Angeles 1959, p. 115.

Grundfest F., An electrophysiological basis of neuropharmacology. Feder. Proc. 17 : 1006, 1958.

Guminska M., Rola α-glicerofosforana v metabolizme węglowodanowym komórok. Post. Biochemii 7 : 499, 1961.

Hager H., Die feinere Cytologie und Cytopathologie des Nervensystems dargestellt auf Grund elektronenmikroskopischer Befunde. G. Fischer Verlag, Stuttgart 1964.

Hager H., Luh S., Ruščáková D. and Ruščák M., Histochemische, elektronenmikroskopische und biochemische Untersuchungen über Glykogenanhäufung in reaktiv veränderten Astrozyten der traumatisch lädierten Säugergrosshirnrinde. Z. Zellforsch. 83 : 295, 1967.

Häkkinen H. M. and Kulonen M., Increase of γ-aminobutyric acid content of rat brain after ingestion of ethanol. Nature 184 : 726, 1959.

Hamberger C. A. and Hydén H., Production of nucleoproteins in the vestibular ganglion. Acta otolaryng. (Stockholm) 75 : 53, 1949.

van Harreveld A., Compounds in brain extracts causing spreading depression of cerebral cortical activity and contraction of crustacean muscle. J. Neurochem. 3 : 300, 1959.

van Harreveld A. and Crowell J., Extracellular space in central nervous tissue. Feder. Proc. 23 : 304, 1964.

van Harreveld A., Crowell J. and Malhotra S. K., A study of extracellular space in cortical nervous tissue by freeze substitution. J. Cell Biol. 25 : 117, 1965.

van Harreveld A. and Khattab F., Changes in cortical extracellular space during spreading depression investigated with the electron microscope. J. Neurophysiol. 30 : 911, 1967.

van Harreveld A. and Kooiman M., Amino acid release from the cerebral cortex during spreading depression and asphyxiation. J. Neurochem. 12 : 431, 1965.

van Harreveld A. and Ochs S., Cerebral impedance changes after circulatory arrest. Amer. J. Physiol. 187 : 180, 1956.

Hartmann J. F., High sodium content of cortical astrocytes. Arch. Neurol. 15 : 633, 1966.

159

Haymaker W. and Strughold H., Atmospheric hypoxidosis. In: Handbuch der speziellen pathologischen Anatomie und Histologie. XIII/1B. Springer, Berlin-Göttingen-Heidelberg 1957, p. 1673.

Heller I. H. and Elliot K. A. C., The metabolism of normal brain and gliomas in relation to cell type and density. Canad. J. Biochem. Physiol. 33 : 395, 1955.

Hempling H. G., Source of energy for the transport of potassium and sodium across the membrane of the Ehrlich mouse ascites tumor cells. Biochim. biophys. Acta 112 : 503, 1966.

Herbert J. D., Coulson R. A. and Hernandez T., Free amino acids in the caiman and rat. Com. Biochem. Physiol. 17 : 583, 1966.

Hertz L., Possible role of neuroglia: a potassium mediated neuronal-neuroglial-neuronal impulse transmission system. Nature 206 : 1091, 1965.

Hertz L., Neuroglial localisation of potassium and sodium effects on respiration in brain. J. Neurochem. 13 : 1373, 1966.

Hertz L. and Clausen T., Effects of potassium and sodium on respiration: their specificity to slices from certain brain regions. Biochem. J. 89 : 526, 1963.

Hertz L. and Schou M., Univalent cations and the respiration of brain cortex slices. Biochem. J. 85 : 93, 1962.

Hess B., Koordination von Atmung und Glykolyse. In: Funktionelle und morphologische Organisation der Zelle. Springer Verlag, Berlin-Göttingen-Heidelberg 1963, p. 163.

Hesselbach M. L. and du Buy H. G., Localisation of glycolytic and respiratory enzyme systems in isolated mouse brain mitochondria. Proc. Soc. exp. Biol. Med. 83 : 62, 1953.

Hillarp A., Cell reactions in hypothalamus following overloading in the antidiuretic function. Acta endocrinol. (Copenh.) 2 : 33, 1949.

Hillmann H. H. and McIlwain H., Membrane potentials in mammalian cerebral tissue in vitro: dependence on ionic environment. J. Physiol. 157 : 263, 1961.

Hindmarsh J. T., Kilby D. and Wiseman G., Effect of amino acids on sugar absorption. J. Physiol. 186 : 166, 1966.

Hochberg J. and Hydén H., The cytochemical correlate of motor nerve cells in spastic paralysis. Acta physiol. scand. 17, suppl. 60 : 1, 1949.

Hodgkin A. L. and Horowitz P., Movements of Na^+ and K^+ in single muscle fibres. J. Physiol. 145 : 40, 1959.

Hodgkin A. L. and Keynes R. D., The potassium permeability of a giant nerve fibre. J. Physiol. 128 : 61, 1955.

Hoffman J. F., Molecular mechanisms of active cation transport. In: Biophysics of Physiological and Pharmacological Actions. Washington, Amer. Association for the Advancement of Science 1961, p. 49.

Hogeboom G. H. and Schneider W. C., Intracellular distribution of enzymes. XI. Glutamic dehydrogenase. J. biol. Chem. 204 : 233, 1953.

Hohorst H. J., Kreutz F. H. and Bücher Th., Über Metabolitgehalte und Metabolitkonzentration in der Leber der Ratte. Biochem. Z. 332 : 18, 1959.

Honour A. J. and McLennan H., The effects of γ-aminobutyric acid and other compounds on structures of the mammalian nervous system which are inhibited by Factor I. J. Physiol. 150 : 306, 1960.

Hook R. H. and Vestling C. S., The two forms of rat-liver aspartate transaminase. Biochem. biophys. Acta 65 : 358, 1962.

Hopper S. and Segal H. L., Comparative properties of glutamic-alanine transaminase from several sources. Arch. Biochem. Biophys. 105 : 501, 1964.

Howe H. A. and Bodian D., Refractoriness of nerve cells to poliomyelitis virus after interruption of their axones. Bull. John Hopkins Hosp. 69 : 92, 1951.

Huijing F. and Slater E. C., The use of oligomycin as an inhibitor of oxidative phosphorylation. J. Biochem. (Jap.) 49 : 493, 1961.

Huxley A. F., Die quantitative Analyse der Nervenerregung und Nervenleitung. Angew. Chemie 76 : 668, 1964.

Hydén H., Protein metabolism of the nerve cell during growth and function. Acta physiol. scandinav. 6, suppl. 17 : 1, 1943.

Hydén, H. The Neuron. In: The Cell. Ed. by J. Brachet and A. E. Mirsky, Acad. Press, New York-London 1960, p. 215.

Ireverre F., Evans R. L., Hayden A. R. and Silber R., Occurence of γ-guanidinobutyric acid. Nature 180 : 704, 1957.

Ito K., Metabolic relationship of succinate and pyruvate in brain tissue with special reference to the potassium effect. Jap. J. exp. Med. 30 : 261, 1960.

Iyer G. J. N. and Sukumaram N., Some studies on transamination with oxalacetate. Canad. J. Biochem. Physiol. 37 : 1517, 1959.

Jacob A., Normale und pathologische Anatomie und Histologie des Grossgehirns. Teil I. Thieme, Leipzig-Vienna 1927.

Jasper H., Gonzales S. and Elliot K. A. C., Action of γ-aminobutyric acid and strychnine upon evoked electrical responses of cerebral cortex. Feder. Proc. 17 : 79, 1958.

Jasper H. H., Khan R. T. and Elliot K. A. C., Amino acids released from the cerebral cortex in relation to its state of activation. Science 147 : 1448, 1965.

Johnsson M. K., The intracellular distribution of glycolytic and other enzymes in rat brain homogenates and mitochondrial preparations. Biochem. J. 77 : 610, 1960.

Johnsson M. K., Inactivation of anaerobic glycolysis in fractions of rat brain homogenates. Biochem. J. 82 : 281, 1962.

Johnston V. P. and Roots B. I., The neurone surface. Nature 205 : 778, 1965.

Judah J. D. and Ahmed K., The biochemistry of sodium transport. Biol. Rev. 39 : 160, 1964.

Kaplanskiy S. Ya. and Berezovskaya N. N., Sintez alanina iz pirovinogradnoy kisloty i ammiaka ochischennym fermentnym preparatom iz mitochondriy pecheni krys. Biokhimiya 23 : 669, 1958.

Katzmann R., Electrolyte distribution in mammalian central nervous system: Are glia high sodium cells? Neurology 11 : 27, 1961.

van Kempen G. M. J., van den Berg C. J., van der Helm H. J. and Veldstra H., Intracellular localisation of glutamatdecarboxylase, γ-aminobutyrate transaminase and some other enzymes in brain tissue. J. Neurochem. 12 : 581, 1965.

Kerr S. E., The carbohydrate metabolism of the brain. I. The determination of glycogen in nerve tissue. J. biol. Chem. 116 : 1, 1936.

Kety S. S., The general metabolism of the brain in vivo. In: Metabolism of the Nervous System. Ed. by D. Richter, Pergamon Press, New York-London 1957, p. 221.

Keynes R. D. and Lewis P. R., The resting exchange of radioactive potassium in crab nerve. J. Physiol. 114 : 151, 1951.

Killam K. F., Convulsants hydrazides. II. Comparison of electrical changes and enzyme inhibition induced by the administration of thiosemicarbazide. J. Pharmacol. 119 : 263, 1957.

Killam K. F., Possible role of γ-aminobutyric acid as an inhibitory transmitter. Feder. Proc. 17 : 1018, 1958.

Kini M. M. and Quastel J. H., Carbohydrate-amino acids interrelations in brain in vitro. Nature 184 : 252, 1959.

Klatzo I. J., Miquel C. I. and Haymaker W., Effect of the alpha-particle irradiation on brain glycogen in the rat. J. Neurochem. 9 : 213, 1962.

Klein E. E., Glutaminovaya kislota v obmene veschestv golovnogo mozga. Usp. sovr. Biol. 41 : 161, 1956.

Klein R. J. and Olsen N. S., Effect of convulsive activity upon the concentration of brain glucose, glycogen, lactate and phosphate. J. biol. Chem. 167 : 747, 1947.

Kleinzeller A., Cyklus kyseliny citronové v látkové přeměně. Čs. fysiol. 3 : 315, 1954.

Kleinzeller A. and Rybová R., Glycogen synthesis in brain cortex slices and some factors affecting it. J. Neurochem. 2 : 45, 1957.

Klingenberg M., Struktur und funktionelle Biochemie der Mitochondrien. II. Die funktionelle Biochemie der Mitochondrien. In: Funktionelle und morphologische Organisation der Zelle. Springer Verlag, Berlin-Göttingen-Heidelberg 1963, p. 69.

Koch A., Rank B. and Newman L., Ionic content of neuroglia. Exp. Neurol. 1 : 186, 1962.

Koeppe R. E. and Hahn Ch. H., Concerning pyruvate metabolism in rat brain. J. biol. Chem. 237 : 1026, 1962.

Kometiani P. A., Svyaz prevrascheniy aminokislot s obmenom ammiaka v golovnom mozgu. Ukr. biokh. Zh. 37 : 721, 1965.

Korey S. R. and Orchen M., Relative respiration of neuronal and glial cells. J. Neurochem. 3 : 277, 1959.

Kornberg A., Lactic dehydrogenase of muscle. In: Methods of Enzymology, vol. I. Ed. by S. P. Colowick and N. O. Kaplan, Acad. Press, New York 1955, p. 441.

Krebs H. A., Metabolism of amino acids. III. Deamination of amino acids. Biochem. J. 28 : 1620, 1935.

Krebs H. A., Body size and tissue respiration. Biochim. biophys. Acta 4 : 249, 1950.

Krebs H. A. and Bellamy D., The interconversion of glutamic acid and aspartic acid in respiring tissues. Biochem. J. 75 : 523, 1960.

Krieg W. J. S., Connections of the cerebral cortex. I. The albino rat. J. compar. Neurol. 84 : 221, 1946.

Kritzmann M. G., Über den Ab- und Aufbau von Aminosäuren durch Umaminierung. Enzymologia 5 : 44, 1938.

Krnjevic K. and Schwartz S., The action of γ-aminobutyric acid on cortical neurons. Exp. Brain Res. 3 : 320, 1967.

Křivánek J., Changes of brain glycogen in the spreading EEG depression of Leão. J. Neurochem 2 : 337, 1957.

Křivánek J., Inkorporace ^{35}P do fosforečných frakcí krysího mozku při šířící se EEG depresi Čs. fysiol. 8 : 417, 1959.

Křivánek J., Some metabolic changes accompanying Leão's spreading cortical depression in the rat. J. Neurochem. 6 : 183, 1961.

Křivánek J., Concerning the dynamics of the metabolic changes accompanying cortical spreading depression. Physiol. bohemoslov. 11 : 383, 1962.

Křivánek J. and Bureš J., K některým metabolickým aspektům šířící se EEG deprese. Čs. fysiol. 7 : 497, 1958.

Křivánek J. and Bureš J., Význam draselných iontů pro šíření šířící se deprese. Čs. fysiol. 9 : 437, 1960.

Křivánek J., Bureš J. and Burešová O., Evidence for relation between creatine phosphate level and polarity of the cerebral cortex. Nature 182 : 1799, 1958.

Kuffler S. W. and Nicholls J. G., The physiology of neuroglial cells. Erg. Physiol. 57 : 1, 1966.

Kulenkampf H., Das Verhalten der Vorderwurzelzellen der weissen Maus unter dem Reiz physiologischer Tätigkeit. Z. Anat. Entwicklgesch. 116 : 143, 1951.

Kuriyama K., Roberts E. and Rubinstein M. K., Elevation of γ-aminobutyric acid in brain with aminooxyacetic acid and susceptibility to convulsive seizures in mice: a quantitative re-evaluation. Biochem. Pharmacol. 15 : 22, 1966.

Lajtha A., Berl E. and Waelsch H., Amino acid and protein metabolism of the brain. IV. The metabolism of glutamic acid. J. Neurochem. 3 : 322, 1959.

Landström H., Caspersson T. and Wohlfart G., Über den Nukleotidumsatz der Nervenzelle. Z. mikr. anat. Forsch. 49 : 534, 1941.

Lardy H. A. and Parks R. E. jr., Enzymes: Units of biological structure and function. Ed. by O. H. Gaebler, Acad. Press, New York 1956, p. 584.

Lardy H. A., Johnson D. and McMurray W. C., Antibiotics as tools for metabolism study. A survey of toxic antibiotics as respiratory and phosphorylative poisons in glycolytic systems. Arch. Biochem. Biophys. 78 : 587, 1958.

Larsen O. and Kjaer A., Paper chromatographic differentiation between L-amino acids and other ninhydrinpositive substances. Biochim. biophys. Acta 38 : 148, 1960.

Lindau O., Quastel J. H. and Sved S., Biochemical studies on chlorpromazine. II. Effects of chlorpromazine on incorporation into proteins and breakdown of glycine 1-^{14}C by isolated rat brain cortex. Canad. J. Biochem. Physiol. 35 : 1145, 1957.

Lindsay H. A. and Barr M. L., Further observations on the behaviour of nuclear structures during depletion and restoration of Nissl material. J. Anat. (Lond.) 89 : 47, 1955.

Lolley R. N., The calcium content of isolated cerebral tissues and their steady-state exchange of calcium. J. Neurochem. 10 : 665, 1963.

de Lores Arnaiz G. R., Alberici M. and de Robertis E., Ultrastructural and enzymic studies of cholinergic and noncholinergic synaptic membranes isolated from brain cortex. J. Neurochem. 14 : 215, 1967.

de Lores Arnaiz G. R. and de Robertis E., 5-Hydroxytryptophane decarboxylase activity in nerve endings of the rat brain. J. Neurochem. 11 : 213, 1964.

Løvtrup S., The subcellular localisation of glutamic acid decarboxylase in rat brain. J. Neurochem. 8 : 243, 1961.

Løvtrup S. and Zelander T., Isolation of brain mitochondria. Exp. Cell Res. 27 : 468, 1962.

Lowry O. H., Quantitative Analysis of Single Nerve Cell Bodies. In: Ultrastructure and Cellular Chemistry of Neural Tissue. Ed. by H. Waelsch, New York 1957, p. 69.

Lukyanova L. and Bureš J., Změny pO$_2$ vyvolávané šířící se depresí v kůře a nucleus caudatus krysy. Čs. fysiol. 16 : 263, 1967.

Luse S. A., Electron microscopic observation of the central nervous system. J. biophys. biochem. Cytol. 2 : 531, 1956.

Machiyama Y., Balázs R. and Julian I., Oxidation of glucose through the γ-aminobutyrate pathway in brain. Biochem. J. 96 : 60P, 1965.

Marshall W. H., Spreading cortical depression. Physiol. Rev. 39 : 239, 1959.

Martin J. B. and Doty D. M., Determination of inorganic phosphate. Analyt. Chem. 21 : 965, 1949.

Maslova M. N. and Rozengart V. I., Soderzhaniye γ-aminomaslyanoy kisloty v mozgu razlichnykh zhivotnykh pri sudorogakh. Tretya vsesoyuznaya konferentsiya po biokhimii nervnoy sistemy. AN ASSR, Erevan 1963, p. 153.

Massieu G. H., Ortega B. G., Syrquin A. and Tuena M., Free amino acids in brain and liver of deoxipyridoxine treated mice subjected to insulin shock. J. Neurochem. 9 : 143, 1962.

Maxwell D. S. and Kruger L., The fine structure of astrocytes in the cerebral cortex and their response to focal injury produced by heavy ionizing particles. J. Cell Biol. 25 : 141, 1965.

Maynard E. A., Schultz R. L. and Pease D. C., Electron microscopy of the vascular bed of rat cerebral cortex. Amer. J. Anat. 100 : 409, 1957.

McDonald R. E. and Waterbury W. E., Colorimetric estimation of citric acid. Nature 184 : 988, 1959.

McIlwain H., Biochemistry and the Central Nervous System. Churchill Ltd., London 1959.

McKhann G. M., Albers R. W., Sokoloff L., Mickelsen O. and Tower D. B., The quantitative significance of the gamma-aminobutyric acid pathway in cerebral oxidative metabolism. In: Inhibition in the Central Nervous System and Gamma-aminobutyric acid. Ed. by E. Roberts, Pergamon Press, Oxford-London-New York-Paris 1960, p. 169.

McKhann G. M. and Tower D. B., Gamma-aminobutyric acid: a substrate for oxidative metabolism of cerebral cortex. Amer. J. Physiol. 196 : 36, 1959.

McKhann G. M. and Tower D. B., The regulation of γ-aminobutyric acid metabolism in cerebral cortex mitochondria. J. Neurochem. 7 : 26, 1961.

McLennan H., Absence of γ-aminobutyric acid from brain extracts containing Factor I. Nature 181 : 1807, 1958.

McLennan H., The identification of one active component from brain extracts containing Facto I. J. Physiol. 146 : 358, 1959.

Meister A., Transamination in amino acid metabolism. Feder. Proc. 14 : 683, 1955.

Meister A., Metabolism of glutamine. Physiol. Rev. 46 : 103, 1956.

Mikeš O., Descendentní papírová elektroforese bílkovinných hydrolyzátů a peptidů. Chem. listy 51 : 138, 1957.

Minikami S., Kakinuma K. and Yoshikawa H., The control of respiration in brain slices. Biochim. biophys. Acta 78 : 808, 1963.

Miquel J. and Haymaker W., Astroglial reaction to ionizing radiation: with emphasis on glycogen accumulation. In: Biology of Neuroglia. Ed. by E. D. P. de Robertis and A. Carrea, Elsevier, Amsterdam 1965, p. 89.

Miquel J., Klatzo I., Menzel D. B. and Haymaker W., Glycogen changes in x-irradiated rat brain. Acta neuropath. 2 : 482, 1963.

Moore S. and Stein W. H., Procedures for the chromatographic determination of amino acids on four per cent cross linked sulphonated polystyren resins. J. biol. Chem. 211 : 893, 1954.

Mori A., Influence of γ-aminobutyric acid and substances possessing similar chemical structure on hexokinase of the brain and heart muscle. J. Biochem. (Jap.) 45 : 985, 1958.

Morlock N. L., Mori K. and Ward A. A. jr., A study of single cortical neurons during spreading depression. J. Neurophysiol. 27 : 1192, 1964.

Mullins L. J., Substrate utilisation by stimulated nerve. Amer. J. Physiol. 175 : 358, 1953.

Nechaeva G., Khod obnovleniya sery belkov, glyutationa i sulfatidov golovnogo mozga krys v sostoyaniyi narkoticheskogo sna i pri vozbuzhdenii centralnoy nervnoy sistemy. Biokhimiya 22 : 546, 1957.

Newsholme E. A., Randle P. J. and Manchester K. L., Inhibition of the phosphofructokinase reaction in perfused rat heart by respiration of ketone bodies, fatty acids and pyruvates. Nature 193 : 270, 1962.

Nurnberger J. I., Direct enumeration of cells of the brain. In: Biology of Neuroglia. Ed. by F. W. Windle, Ch. C. Thomas, Springfield, Ill. 1958, p. 193.

Oksche A., Histologische Untersuchungen über die Bedeutung des Ependyms, der Glia und der Plexus chlorioidei für den Kohlehydratstoffwechsel des ZNS. Z. Zellforsch. 48 : 74, 1958.

Oksche A., Der histochemisch nachweisbare Glykogenaufbau und Abbau in den Astrozyten und Ependymzellen als Beispiel einer funktionsabhängigen Stoffwechselaktivität der Neuroglia. Z. Zellforsch. 54 : 307, 1961.

Okumura N., Otsuki S. and Nasu H., The influence of insulin hypoglycaemic coma, repeated electroshocks and chlorpromazine or β-phenylisopropylmethylamine administration on the free amino-acids in the brain. J. Biochem. (Jap.) 46 : 247, 1959.

O'Neil J. J., Simon S. H. and Skreewe W. W., Alternate glycolytic pathway in brain. A comparison between the action of artificial electron acceptors and electrical stimulation. J. Neurochem. 12 : 979, 1965.

Palladin A. V., Biokhimicheskaya kharakteristika funkcionalnogo sostoyaniya razlichnykh otdelov nervnoy sistemy. Ukr. biokh. Zh. 31 : 765, 1959.

Palladin A. V., Belik Ya. V. and Krachko L. S., Skorost obnovleniya belkov v mozgu pri vozbuzhdeniyi i tormozheniyi i v zavisomosti ot vozrasta zhivotnogo. Biokhimiya 22 : 359, 1957.

Palladin A. V., Belik Ya. V. and Krachko L. S., Vnedreniye metionina ^{35}S v belki razlichnykh strukturnykh elementov kletok polushariy golovnogo mozga. Dokl. Akad. Nauk SSSR 127 : 702, 1959.

Passonneau J. V. and Lowry O. H., Phosphofructokinase and the regulation of glycolysis. Feder. Proc. 21 : 87, 1962.

Peters R. A., Pyruvate metabolism in the central nervous system. In: Neurochemistry. Ed. by K. A. C. Elliot, Ch. C. Thomas, Springfield, Ill. 1955, p. 111.

Petrushka E. and Giuditta A., Electron microscopy of two subcellular fractions isolated from cerebral cortex homogenates. J. biochem. biophys. Cytol. 6 : 129, 1959.

Pevzner L. Z., Soderzhaniye citoplasmaticheskoy RNK v neyronakh raznykh kletochnykh sloyev kory golovnogo mozga v norme i pri gipoksiyi. Tretya vsesoyuznaya konf. po biokhimiyi nervnoy sistemy. AN ASSR, Erevan 1963, p. 327.

di Pietro D. and Weinhouse S., Glucose oxidation in rat brain slices and homogenates. Arch. Biochem. Biophys. 80 : 268, 1959.

Porcelatti G. and Thompson R. H. S., The effect of nerve section on the free amino acids in nervous tissue. J. Neurochem. 1 : 340, 1957.

Price G. M., The accumulation of α-alanine in the housefly Musca vicina. Biochem. J. 81 : 15P 1961.

Price G. M. and Moriyua S., Effects of anoxia on the metabolism of amino acids by the adult housefly (musca domestica) in vivo. Biochem. J. 84 : 98P, 1962.

Prokhorova N. I. and Tupikova Z. N., Intenzivnost obmena uglevodov v organakh pri razlichnykh funkcionalnykh sostoyaniyakh v organizmakh. In: Uglevody i uglevodnye obmeny v zhivotnom i rastitelnom organizmakh. Izd. Akad. Nauk SSSR, Moscow 1959, p. 120.

Purpura D. P., Girado M., Smith T. G. and Gomez J. A., Synaptic effects of systemic γ-aminobutyric acid in cortical regions of increased vascular permeability. Proc. Soc. exp. Biol. Med. 79 : 348, 1958.

Pyatnickaya I. N., O sinteze aminokislot iz ketokislot i ammoniynykh soley v pochkakh krys. Biokhimiya 25 : 86, 1960.

Quastel J. H., Enzymatic mechanisms of the brain and the effects of some neurotropic agents . In: Biochemistry of the Central Nervous System. Ed. by F. Bruecke, Pergamon Press, New York-London-Paris-Los Angeles 1959, p. 90.

Quastel J. H., Molecular transport at cell membranes. Proc. Roy. Soc. B. 163 : 169, 1965.

Quastel J. H. and Quastel D. M. J., The Chemistry of Brain Metabolism in Health and Disease. Ch. C. Thomas, Springfield, Ill, 1961, p. 9.

Reed D. J. and Woodbury D. M., Kinetics of ^{14}C sucrose distribution in cerebral cortex. Cerebrospinal fluid and plasma of rats. Feder. Proc. 19 : 80, 1960.

Reynolds E. S., The use of lead citrate at high pH as an electron opaque stain in electron microscopy. J. Cell Biol. 17 : 208, 1963.

Richter D., Protein metabolism of the brain. In: Biochemistry of the Central Nervous System. Ed. by F. Bruecke, Pergamon Press, New York-London-Paris-Los Angeles 1959, p. 173.

Richter D. and Dawson R. M. C., Brain metabolism in emotional excitement and sleep. Amer. J. Physiol. 154 : 73, 1948.

Ridge J. W., Resting and stimulated respiration in vitro in the central nervous system. Regional distribution and relation to cell density. Biochem. J. 105 : 831, 1967.

Rindi G. and Ferrari G., The γ-aminobutyric acid and glutamic acid content of brains of rats treated with toxopyrimidine. Nature 183 : 608, 1959.

Rixon R. H. and Whitfield J. F., The effect of elevated salt concentrations on the nuclear structures of L-mouse cells. Exp. Cell Res. 26 : 591, 1962.

de Robertis E., Ultrastructure and cytochemistry of the synaptic region. Science 156 : 907, 1967.

de Robertis E., de Iraldi A. P., Arnaiz de Lores G. R. and Salganicoff L., Cholinergic and non-cholinergic nerve endings in rat brain. I. Isolation and subcellular distribution of acetylcholinesterase. J. Neurochem. 9 : 23, 1962.

de Robertis E., Sellinger O. Z., de Lores Arnaiz G. R., Alberici M. and Zicher L. M., Nerve endings in methionine sulfoximine convulsant rats; a neurochemical and ultrastructural study. J. Neurochem. 14 : 81, 1967.

de Robertis E. D. P., Some new electron microscopical contributions to the biology of neuroglia. In: Biology of Neuroglia. Ed. by E. D. P. de Robertis and A. Carrea, Elsevier, Amsterdam 1965, p. 1.

Roberts E., Free amino acids of nervous tissues. Some aspects of metabolism of gamma-aminobutyric acid. In: Inhibition in the Central Nervous System and Gamma-Aminobutyric Acid. Ed. by E. Roberts, Pergamon Press, Oxford-London-New York-Paris 1960, p. 144.

Roberts E. and Baxter C. F., γ-Aminobutyric acid in brain: its formation from glutamic acid. J. biol. Chem. 187 : 55, 1960.

Roberts E. and Baxter C. F., γ-Aminobutyric acid in brain. In: Biochemistry of the Central Nervous System. Ed. by F. Bruecke, Pergamon Press, London-New York-Paris-Los Angeles 1959, p. 268.

Roberts E. and Bregoff H. M., Transamination of γ-aminobutyric acid and β-alanine in brain and liver. J. biol. Chem. 201 : 393, 1953.

Roberts E., Flexner J. B. and Flexner L. B., Biochemical and physiological differentiation during morphogenesis. XXIII. Further observations relating to the synthesis of amino acids and proteins by the cerebral cortex and liver of the mouse. J. Neurochem. 4 : 78, 1959.

Roberts E., Frankel S. and Harman J. P., Amino acids of nervous tissue. Proc. Soc. exp. Biol. Med. 74 : 383, 1950.

Roberts E. and Kuriyama K., Biochemical-physiological correlations in studies of the γ-aminobutyric acid system. Brain Res. 8 : 1, 1968.

Roberts E., Lowe I. P., Guth L. and Jelinek B., Distribution of γ-aminobutyric acid and other amino acids in nervous tissue of various species. J. exp. Zool. 128 : 313, 1958.

Roberts E., Rothstein M. and Baxter C. F., Some metabolic studies of γ-aminobutyric acid. Proc. Soc. exp. Biol. Med. 97 : 796, 1958.

Robinson H. E., Gamma aminobutyric acid and brain metabolism. Nutr. Rev. 17 : 278, 1959.

Roots B. I. and Johnston P. V., Neurons of ox brain nuclei: their isolation and appearance by light and electron microscopy. J. Ultrastr. Res. 10 : 350, 1964.

de Ropp R. S. and Snedeker E. H., Effect of drugs on amino acid levels in the rat brain: hypoglycemic agents. J. Neurochem. 7 : 128, 1961.

de Ropp R. S. and Snedeker E. H., Sequential one dimensional chromatography: analysis of free amino acids in the brain. Analyt. Biochem. 1 : 424, 1960.

Rose S. P. R., Preparation of enriched fractions from cerebral cortex containing isolated, metabolically active neuronal and glial cells. Biochem. J. 102 : 33, 1967.

Rossiter N., Lipid metabolism. In: Metabolism of the Nervous System. Ed. by D. Richter, Pergamon Press, London-New York-Paris-Los Angeles 1957, p. 267.

van Rossum G. D. V., The effect of oligomycin on net movements of sodium and potassium in mammalian cells in vitro. Biochim. biophys. Acta 82 : 556, 1964.

Rothstein A., Membrane phenomena. Ann. Rev. Physiol. 30 : 15, 1968.

du Ruisseau J. P., Greenstein J. P., Winitz M. and Birnbaum S. M., Studies on the metabolism of amino acids and related compounds in vivo. VI. Free amino acid levels in the tissues of rats protected against ammonia toxicity. Arch. Biochem. Biophys. 68 : 161, 1957.

Rummel W., Seifen E. and Baldauf J., Influence of calcium and ouabain upon the potassium efflux in human erythrocytes. Biochem. Pharmacol. 12 : 557, 1963.

Ruščák M., Ein Beitrag zum Gehirnmetabolismus bei EEG Depression. Biológia 15 : 460, 1960.

Ruščák M., Über die bedingte Reaktion auf den erhöhten Muskelstoffwechsel. SAV, Bratislava 1961.

Ruščák M., Changes in amino nitrogen during EEG depression. J. Neurochem. 57 : 305, 1961.

Ruščák M., Influence of various stimuli on lactic acid, alanine and γ-aminobutyric acid levels in rat brains. Nature 195 : 290, 1962.

Ruščák M., Kyselina μ-amínomaslová a jej vzťah k EEG aktivite mozgovej kôry. Čs. fysiol. 12 : 334, 1963.

Ruščák M. and Duda P., K metabolizmu mozgu pri EEG depresii za anémie mozgu. Čs. fysiol. 8 : 429, 1959.

Ruščák M. and Macejová E., Formation of L-α-Alanine and γ-aminobutyric acid in rat cortical slices in relation to the substrate and the pH in the medium. Physiol. bohemoslov. 14 : 266, 1965.

Ruščák M., Macejová E. and Ruščáková D., Porovnanie dýchania a glykolýzy v rezoch a mitochondriách mozgovej kôry krýs. Čs. fysiol. 12 : 334, 1963.

Ruščák M., Macejová E. and Ruščáková D., Effect of L-glutamic and γ-aminobutyric acid on glycolysis in slices and mitochondria of the rat central nervous system. Physiol. bohemoslov. 13 : 156, 1964.

Ruščák M., Macejová E., Ruščáková D. and Mrena E., O glikolize v mitochondriyalnoy fraktsiyi centralnoy nervnoy sistemy krys. Ukr. biokh. Zh. 36 : 584, 1964.

Ruščák M., Ruščáková D. and Hager H., K metabolizmu neurocytov a reaktívnej glie v mozgovej kôre potkanov. Čs. fysiol. 16 : 260, 1967.

Ruščák M., Ruščáková D. and Koníková E., Metabolische Unterschiedlichkeiten zwischen Neurozyten und reaktiver Glia in der Gehirnrinde von Ratten. Biológia 22 : 337, 1967.

Ruščák M., Ruščáková D. and Macejová E., Adenosinetriphosphatase in mitochondrial subfractions of the rat central nervous system and its activation by calcium, magnesium, and manganese ions. Physiol. bohemoslov. 14 : 261, 1965.

Ruščák M. and Whittam R., Vzťah oligomycínu k aktívnemu transportu K^+ iónov rezmi mozgovej kôry králika. Čs. fysiol. 15 : 114, 1966.

Ruščák M. and Whittam R., The metabolic response of brain slices to agents affecting the sodium pump. J. Physiol. 190 : 595, 1967.

Ruščáková D., Über den Einfluss monovalenter Chlorideverbindungen auf die Nervenzellen des zentralen Rindengraus. Biológia 16 : 925, 1961.

Ruščáková D., Effect of potassium ions on the morphological picture of cells of the cerebral cortex. Physiol. bohemoslov. 13 : 161, 1964.

Ruščáková D., Recovery processes in cells of the cerebral cortex after the application of potassium ions. Physiol. bohemoslov. 13 : 167, 1964.

Rybová R., Effect of cations on γ-aminobutyric acid level in slices of brain cortex. Nature 185 : 542, 1960.

Rybová R., The effect of cations on brain cortex metabolism in vitro. In: Membrane Transport and Metabolism. Ed. by A. Kleinzeller and A. Kotyk, Acad. Press Inc., New York 1961, p. 543.

Sachs J. and Morton J. H., Lactic and pyruvic acid relations in contracting mammalian muscle. Amer. J. Physiol. 186 : 221, 1956.

Sacktor B., Regulation of glycolysis in brain, in situ and during convulsions. J. biol. Chem. 241 : 5071, 1966.

Sacktor B., Cummins J. and Packer L., Oxidation of γ-aminobutyrate by brain mitochondria. Feder. Proc. 18 : 314, 1959.

Sacktor B., Packer L. and Estabrook R. W., Respiratory activity of brain mitochondria. Arch. Biochem. Biophys. 80 : 68, 1959.

Sálganicoff L. and de Robertis E. D. P., Subcellular butiidistron of the enzymes of the glutamic acid, glutamine and γ-aminobutyric acid cycles in rat brain. J. Neurochem. 12 : 287, 1965.

Salvador R. A. and Albers R. W., The distribution of glutamic γ-aminobutyric acid transaminase in the nervous system of Rhesus monkey. J. biol. Chem. 234 : 922, 1959.

Schmidt C. G., Gehirn und Nerven. Physiol. Chemie. 20 : 617, 1956.

Schultz R. L., Maynard E. A. and Pease D. C., Electron microscopy of neurons and neuroglia of cerebral cortex and corpus callosum. Amer. J. Anat. 100 : 369, 1957.

Schwartz A., The effect of ouabain on potassium content, phosphoprotein metabolism and oxygen consumption in guinea pig cerebral tissue. Biochem. Pharmacol. 11 : 389, 1962.

Schwartz A. and Lee Kwang Soo, The effect of heart mitochondria on glycolytic systems from brain and heart. Biochim. biophys. Acta 44 : 590, 1960.

Segal H. L., Beattie D. S. and Hopper S., Purification and properties of liver glutamic-alanine transaminase from normal and cortison treated rats. J. biol. Chem. 237 : 1914, 1962.

Seifritz W., The effect of various anaesthetic agents on protoplasm. Anesthesiology 11 : 24, 1951.

Sellinger O. Z., Catanzaro R., Chain E. B. and Pocchiari F., The metabolism of glutamate and aspartate in rat cerebral cortical slices. Proc. Roy. Soc. B. 156 : 148, 1962.

Shatunova N. F. and Sytinski I. A., On the intracellular localisation of glutamate decarboxylase and γ-aminobutyric acid in mammalian brain. J. Neurochem. 11 : 701, 1964.

Shaw R. K. and Heine J. D., Effect of insulin on nitrogenous constituents of rat brain. J. Neurochem. 12 : 527, 1965.

Shimizu N. and Hamuro I., Deposition of glycogen and changes in some enzymes in brain wounds. Nature 181 : 781, 1958.

Shimizu N. and Kubo Z., Histochemical studies on brain glycogen of the guinea pig and its alteration following electric shock. J. Neuropath. 16 : 40, 1957.

Simonoff R. and Saunders P. R., Effect of morphine on the uptake and oxidation of glucose by rabbit brain. J. Neurochem. 5 : 354, 1960.

Skou J. Ch., Further investigations on a $Mg^{++} + Na^+$ activated adenosinetriphosphatase, possibly related to the active, linked transport of Na^+ and K^+ across the nerve membrane. Biochim. biophys. Acta 42 : 6, 1960,

Sokoloff L., Lassen N. A., McKhann G. M., Tower D. B. and Albers W., Effects of pyridoxine with drawal on cerebral circulation and metabolism in a pyridoxine dependent child. Nature 183 : 751, 1959.

Solomon A. K., Red cell membrane structure and ion transport. J. gen. Physiol. 43, suppl. 1, 1960.

Somogyi M., Notes on sugar determination. J. biol. Chem. 195 : 19, 1952.

Steensholt G. and Joner P. S., Some studies in amino acid decarboxylase. Acta chem. scandinav. 11 : 79, 1957.

168

Strecker H. J., Glutamic acid and glutamine. In: Metabolism of the Nervous System. Ed. by D. Richter, Pergamon Press, London-New York 1957, p. 459.

Streicker E., The thiocyanate space in rat brain. Amer. J. Physiol. 201 : 334, 1961.

Svetuchina V. M., Citoarkhitektonika novoy kory mozga v otrasle gryzunov. Arch. Anat. (ZSSR) 42 : 31, 1962.

Swanson P. B. and Clark H. E., The metabolism of proteins and amino acids. Ann. Rev. Biochem. 19 : 235, 1950.

Swick R. S., Barnstein P. J. and Stange J. L., The metabolism of mitochondrial proteins. I. Distribution and characterization of the isozymes of alanine aminotransferase in rat liver. J. biol. Chem. 240 : 3334, 1965.

Šorm F. and Turský T., The effect of anions on the glutamic acid decarboxylase of brain tissue. Coll. Czechoslov. Chem. Commun. 20 : 297, 1955.

Tallan H. H., Moore S. and Stein W. H., Studies on free amino acids and related compounds in the tissues of the cat. J. biol. Chem. 211 : 927, 1954.

Takahashi H., Nagashima H., Koshino Ch. and Takahashi H., Effects of γ-aminobutyric acid (GABA), γ-aminobutyrylcholine and their related substances on the cortical activity. Jap. J. Physiol. 9 : 257, 1959.

Takahashi I. and Abakane J., Protein metabolism of rat brain slices. Canad. J. Biochem. Physiol. 38 : 1149, 1960.

Tanaka R. and Abood L. G., Isolation from rat brain of mitochondria devoid of glycolytic activity. J. Neurochem. 10 : 571, 1963.

Tapia R., Pasantes H., de la Mora M. P., Ortega B. G. and Massieu G. H., Free amino acids and glutamate decarboxylase activity in brain of mice during drug-induced convulsions. Biochem. Pharmacol. 16 : 483, 1967.

Terner C., Eggleston L. V. and Krebs H. A., The role of glutamic acid in the transport of potassium in brain and retina. Biochem. J. 47 : 139, 1950.

Thorn W., Scholl H., Pfleiderer G. and Muelderer B., Stoffwechselvorgänge im Gehirn bei normaler und herabgesetzter Körpertemperatur unter ischämischer und anoxischer Belastung. J. Neurochem. 2 : 150, 1958.

Tigerman H. and McVicar R., Glutamine, glutamic acid and ammonia administration and tissue glutamine. J. biol. Chem. 189 : 793, 1951.

Tobin R. B. and Slater E. C., The effect of oligomycin on the respiration of tissue slices. Biochim. biophys. Acta 105 : 214, 1965.

Torack R. M., The extracellular space of rat brain following perfusion fixation with glutaraldehyde and hydroxyadipealdehyde. Z. Zellforsch. 66 : 352, 1965.

Tower D. B., The neurochemical substrate of cerebral function and activity. In: Biological and Biochemical Bases of Behaviour. Ed. by F. H. Harlow and C. M. Woolseg, Univ. Press of Wisconsin 1958, p. 419.

Tower D. B., Glutamic acid metabolism in the mammalian central nervous system. In: Biochemistry of the Central Nervous System. Ed. by F. Bruecke, Pergamon Press, London-New York-Paris-Los Angeles 1959, p. 213.

Tower D. B., The neurochemistry of asparagine and glutamine. In: The Neurochemistry of Nucleotides and Amino Acids. John Wiley and Sons Inc., New York-London 1960, p. 173.

Tower D. B., The evidence for a neurochemical basis of seizures. In: Temporal Lobe Epilepsy. Ch. C. Thomas, Springfield, Ill. 1958, p. 301.

Troickaya V. B., Vliyaniye [uslovnoreflektornogo vozbuzhdeniya centralnoy nervnoy sistemy na uglevodnofosfornyy obmen v bolshikh polushariyakh golovnogo mozga. Vopr. med. Chim. 4 : 17, 1957.

Tsukada J., Hirano S., Nagati J. and Matsutani T., Metabolic studies of gamma-aminobutyric acid in mammalian tissues. In: Inhibition in the Central Nervous System and Gamma - Aminobutyric acid. Ed. by E. Roberts, Pergamon Press, Oxford-London-New York-Paris 1960, p. 163.

Tsukada J., Nagato J., Hirano S. and Takagaki G., Glucose metabolism and amino acids in brain slices. J. Biochem. (Jap.) 45 : 979, 1958.

Tursky T., Effect of potassium cyanide poisoning on the γ-aminobutyric acid level in the brain. Nature 187 : 322, 1960.

Udenfriend S., Identification of γ-aminobutyric acid in brain by the isotope derivative method. J. biol. Chem. 187 : 65, 1950.

Udenfriend S., Weissbach H. and Mitoma Ch., Metabolism of amino acids. Ann. Rev. Biochem. 29 : 207, 1960.

Utley J. D., The effect of anthranilic hydroxamic acid on rat behaviour and rat brain γ-aminobutyric acid, norepinephrine and 5-hydroxytryptamine concentration. J. Neurochem. 10 : 423, 1963.

Waelsch H., Glutamic acid and cerebral function. Adv. Prot. Chem. 6 : 301, 1951.

Waelsch H., Metabolism of glutamic acid and glutamine. In: Metabolism of the Nervous System. Ed. by D. Richter, Pergamon Press, London-New York 1957, p. 24.

Waelsch H., Some problems of metabolism in relation to the structure of the nervous system. In: Biochemistry of the Central Nervous System. Ed. by F. Bruecke, Pergamon Press, London-New York 1959, p. 36.

Waelsch H. and Lajtha A., Protein metabolism of the nervous system. In: The Neurochemistry of Nucleotides and Amino Acids. John Wiley and Sons Inc., New York-London 1960, p. 205.

Wallach D. P. and Crittenden N. J., Studies on the GABA pathway. I. The inhibition of γ-aminobutyric acid — α-ketoglutaric acid transaminase in vitro and in vivo by U 7524 (aminooxyacetic acid). Biochem. Pharmacol 5 : 323, 1961.

Weil-Malherbe H., Studies on brain metabolism. III. The anaerobic dismutation of α-keto acids. Biochem. J. 31 : 2202, 1937.

Weil-Malherbe H., Observations on tissue glycolysis. Biochem. J. 38 : 2257, 1938.

Weil-Malherbe H., Significance of glutamic acid for the metabolism of nervous tissue. Physiol. Rev. 30 : 549, 1950.

Weil-Malherbe H., L'ammoniaque dans le métabolism cérébral. Schweiz. Med. Wschr. 86 : 1223, 1956.

Wendel-Smith C. P. and Blunt M. J., Possible role of neuroglia. Nature 208 : 600, 1965.

Whisler K. E., Tews J. K. and Stone W. E., Cerebral amino acids and lipids in drug-induced status epilepticus. J. Neurochem. 15 : 215, 1968.

Whittaker W. P., The isolation and characterisation of acetylcholine-containing particles from brain. Biochem. J. 72 : 694, 1959.

Whittaker W. P., The application of subcellular fractionation techniques to the study of brain function. In: Progress in Biophysics and Molecular Biology, vol. 15. Pergamon Press, Oxford-London-New York-Paris-Edinburgh-Frankfurt 1965, p. 41.

Whittaker W. P. and Gray E. G., The synapse: biology and morphology. Brit. Med. Bull. 18 : 223, 1962.

Whittam R., The dependence of the respiration of brain cortex on active cation transport. Biochem. J. 82 : 205, 1962.

Whittam R., The interdependence of metabolism and active transport. In: Hoffmann J. F., Cellular Functions of Membrane Transport. Prentice-Hall Inc., New York 1964, p. 184.

Whittam R. and Blond D. M., Respiratory control by an adenosine triphosphatase involved in active transport in brain cortex. Biochem. J. 92 : 147, 1964.

Whittam R., Wheeler K. P. and Blake A., Oligomycin and active transport reactions in cell membranes. Nature 203 : 720, 1964.

Whittam R. and Willis J. S., Ion movements and oxygen consumption in kidney cortex slices. J. Physiol. 168 : 158, 1963.

Williamson J. R., Glycolytic control mechanism. I. Inhibition of glycolysis by acetate and pyruvate in the isolated, perfused rat heart. J. biol. Chem. 240 : 2308, 1965.

Wilson W. E., Hill R. J. and Koeppe R. E., The metabolism of γ-aminobutyric acid 4^{14}-C by intact rats. J. biol. Chem. 234 : 347, 1959.

Wolfe L. S., Klatzo J., Miquel C. T. and Haymaker W., Effect of the alpha-particle irradiation on brain glycogen in the rat. J. Neurochem. 9 : 213, 1962.

Woodbury D. M., Discussion in Biology of Neuroglia. Ed. by W. F. Windle, Ch. C. Thomas, Springfield, Ill. 1958 p. 120.

Woodbury D. M. and Esplin D. W., Neuropharmacology and neurochemistry of anticonvulsant drugs. In: The Effect of Pharmacologic Agents on the Nervous System. Williams, & Wilkins Co., Baltimore 1959, p. 24.

Woodbury D. M. and Vernadakis A., Relation of brain excitability to brain γ-aminobutyric acid concentration. Feder. Proc. 17 : 420, 1958.

Yakovlev N. N., Ocherki po biokhimii sporta. Medgiz, Moscow 1958.

Zachar J. and Ruščák M., K metabolizmu mozgu pri šíriacej sa EEG depresii. Čs. fysiol. 7 : 191, 1958.

Zachar J. and Zacharová D., Mechanizmus vzniku šíriacej sa kortikálnej EEG depresie. SAV, Bratislava 1963.